The Ageless Body

The Ageless Body

How to Hold Back the Years to Achieve a Better Body

Peta Bee and Dr Sarah Schenker

BLOOMSBURY

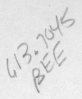
Bloomsbury Sport
An imprint of Bloomsbury Publishing Plc

50 Bedford Square
London
WC1B 3DP
UK

1385 Broadway
New York
NY 10018
USA

www.bloomsbury.com

BLOOMSBURY and the Diana logo are trademarks of Bloomsbury Publishing Plc

First published 2016

© Peta Bee
Diet Plans © Dr Sarah Schenker, 2016
Illustrations @ David Gardner
Photography @ Eddie Macdonald

British Library Cataloguing-in-Publication Data
A catalogue record for this book is available from the British Library.

Library of Congress Cataloguing-in-Publication data has been applied for.

ISBN: PB: 978-1-4729-2441-4
ePDF: 978-1-4729-2443-8
ePub: 978-1-4729-2442-1

4 6 8 10 9 7 5 3

Typeset in Minion by Deanta Global Publishing Services, Chennai, India
Printed and bound in Great Britain by CPI Group (UK) Ltd, Croydon CR0 4YY

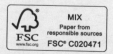

MIX
Paper from
responsible sources
FSC® C020471
FSC
www.fsc.org

To find out more about our authors and books visit www.bloomsbury.com. Here you will find extracts, author interviews, details of forthcoming events and the option to sign up for our newsletters.

Contents

Preface   1

PART ONE

CHAPTER 1:   Introduction   13
CHAPTER 2:   The Science of Ageing   32
CHAPTER 3:   Eating for an Ageless Body   50
CHAPTER 4:   Exercise for an Ageless Body   71
CHAPTER 5:   The Ageless Body and Longevity   94

PART TWO

CHAPTER 6:   How to Use This Book   105
CHAPTER 7:   The Ageless Body Diet Plan   120
CHAPTER 8:   Recipes and Shopping Lists   127
CHAPTER 9:   The Four-Week Ageless Body Exercise Plans   171
CHAPTER 10: The Exercises   210
CHAPTER 11: How to Keep Going   241
CHAPTER 12: Troubleshooter   250

About the Authors   257
References   258
Index   263

Preface

'My ass is definitely higher than it was when I was 20. This is the thing that people don't understand – take care of your body [and it will] get better! It gets better as I get older.'

Cameron Diaz

As I write this my 47th birthday is looming. I'm edging ever closer to the half-century milestone beyond which women once tipped into a matronly state of old age. Photographs of my grand-mothers, who reached their fifties in the 1950s and 1960s, reveal attractive women who had all but given up hope of feeling glamorous again. The waspish waists and coiffed hair of their formative years had given way to thickened middles and a stouter profile; they looked, dressed and behaved 'old'. They adopted a uniform of flat Hush Puppies shoes and Crimplene dresses, a ritual of weekly sets and perms and then got on with it, knowing that society expected no more, no less of them. They withered into female oblivion.

What strikes me when I flick through my family albums is how starkly their perception of ageing and what it should entail, and their willingness to accept and get on with it, differs from how I see myself as a woman of a similar age today. I belong to a generation of 40-, 50- and 60-year-olds who have experienced a seismic shift in attitudes to ageing. A remarkable phenomenon has taken hold: we don't fear getting older, we relish being wiser and more comfortable with who we are and how we feel. A poll of 2000 women revealed the fifties as being the most sex-confident decade of a woman's life

1

and the over-45s spend more on beauty products than any other age group [1]. We look better and feel better than women of our vintage ever did previously.

Don't get me wrong, this new guard of the 40-plus female is not hanging on to youth in desperation. We don't want to be 20 again, neither do we want to live forever. That longing went out with the 1990s, when diets and workouts were about extolling youth, not preserving it. Gone, too, are the chiselled, over-worked midlife bodies that we saw a decade ago, replaced instead by more delicate muscle definition and limbs that are less scrawny, but leaner and lengthier than they appeared even in their twenties.

This emerging breed of mature woman is redefining expectations of the midlife body and proving that seemingly impossible goals are there for the taking. We have our own set of goals, our own set of role models each flaunting exquisite figures that are barely distinguishable from their 30-year-old selves. From Gwen Stefani and Cameron Diaz to Jennifer Aniston and Dame Helen Mirren, they are redefining not just what a midlife body looks like, but what's entailed in achieving it.

Their message is clear: while getting older is inevitable, wallowing in the slowing metabolism and decreased muscle tone it brings is no longer accepted. And with the right approach, you may just be able to hit the pause button. What matters is how you go about defying the years. And the rules have changed. In *The Ageless Body*, our job is to set about redefining them.

WHAT'S CHANGED?

This is not a book about turning back the clock or about anti-ageing as we've come to accept the meaning of the term – via Botox and fillers, stretching and injecting. Not that we are against such procedures, but we believe there are more fulfilling ways to hit the pause button. Neither, for that matter, is it about clinging on to youth in desperation. If you feel the need to starve yourself of carbs, to schedule in five Spinning sessions a week and back-to-back yoga classes alongside training for your first triathlon, it really is not the thing you should be reading.

A dramatic shift in expectations means that, despite being plagued by the slowing metabolism that afflicts all pre- and post-menopausal women, we can realistically aim for a flat stomach and sculpted arms. Diet and exercise needn't leave you looking as ropey and sinewy as the over-worked Sarah Jessica Parker, but it can leave you effortlessly toned, embodying the kind of appearance we all took for granted in our thirties. We can eat without gaining weight (hooray), consume carbs without them heading straight for the stomach and hips. But we need to recalibrate and re-set our systems in order to achieve an Ageless Body and relish the benefits it brings.

In the course of writing this book, Sarah and I have rifled through endless scientific papers, and tapped the world's leading academic ageing experts for insights into what we can do to decelerate the rate at which we look and feel older. We have also used ourselves as guinea pigs. Both in our forties (me towards the top of the age group, Sarah a relative newbie to the decade), we have children, demanding jobs, hectic social lives and little time to devote to much else. In theory, we didn't have time to overhaul our lifestyles, but we made it and the results have been transformational in many ways.

So what have we discovered? In a nutshell, many of the rules you thought held true for diet and exercise are irrelevant from this age onward. We know from our investigations and the emerging science that standard diet and activity advice simply doesn't work from your mid-thirties onwards. What's required is a radical alternative, an approach that has the potential to change the way you eat and exercise forever.

What can you expect? Workouts will be shorter and harder. Endless aerobic activities that were the gym fixation of the last three decades are unnecessary for maintaining and improving fitness as you get older. Indeed, throwing yourself into repetitive marathons and triathlons after 40 is now considered the ageing equivalent of sunbathing. Hugely effective in terms of fat loss, these long, pounding activities can leave you drawn and haggard.

Too much endurance slogging stresses the skin in a way that causes wear and tear and leads to a drop in its youthful plumpness. You still need it – but in shorter bursts. Up to 45 minutes of jogging, cycling or fast walking three times a week – and not going at breakneck speed – could be enough. Scientists at McMaster University in Canada reported that this kind of approach was enough to boost skin plumpness in the outer and inner layers of a group of volunteers aged 65 and older. After three months, the complexion of the exercisers resembled what the scientists said they'd typically expect to find in healthy 20–40-year-olds [2].

You'll need to work harder for a shorter time to get results and we introduce the principles of High Intensity Interval Training (or HIIT): it minimizes the amount of pounding (not good for vulnerable tendons and knees either) but works the heart and boosts metabolism (strictly necessary: it plummets by as much as 25 per cent as we age). And strength training becomes essential. There's little doubt we need it post-35 when muscle begins diminishing at a rate of 1lb (0.5kg) a year leaving you with sag and sinew unless you address it. As someone who'd always feared weights, I am a convert and a firm one (in every way). In fact, none of the workout methods should scare you: be prepared to be won over from the first week.

Your diet will also come under scrutiny. You will be eating less of the foods that detract from healthful vibrancy, more of the stuff that helps to maintain it for longer than women have in the past. Calories will be considerably lower than is recommended for women of our age; snacks are out and the benefits of breakfast are questioned. But we promise you won't go hungry. What's more, you will be brimful of energy, your skin will glow and you will not only look healthier, but feel better from within.

> 'I have absolutely no objection to growing older. I am a stroke survivor so I am extremely grateful to be ageing – I have nothing but gratitude for the passing years. I am ageing – lucky, lucky me!'
>
> Sharon Stone

Peta's background

My love affair with exercise and the science that underpins it is as enduring as Sarah's passion for food. I was always an active child and took up competitive running at primary school, eventually competing for Wales at middle distance and cross-country. My interest in what makes the human body tick, and how we can propel ourselves to physical extremes, led to me studying for a degree in sports science and another in nutrition at university.

Fitness even became the prime focus of my career as a journalist and for more than two decades I have written about sports science, exercise and their impact on health and longevity in *The Times, Daily Mail, Sunday Times, Evening Standard* and many other websites and publications. More recently, I have immersed myself in the highly scientific and technical aspects of fitness for elite sport as performance editor for *Athletics Weekly*. In 2008 and 2012 I was named Medical Journalists' Association's Freelancer of the Year and I have written seven previous books about health and fitness including the bestseller *Fast Exercise* with Dr Michael Mosley of BBC *Horizon* fame.

Much of what I have seen through my work has left me cynical. I've discovered that, much like the diet world, the fitness industry too often bases itself on false promises and faddy workout regimens that hold no water scientifically. What's hot in gyms today will invariably not be making you sweat tomorrow. The more I witnessed, the less inspired I became by what the gym industry had to offer. And the more frustrated I was with the knowledge that people were investing time and money without getting just reward in the shape of a body in which they should be proud. My gut instinct has always been that to get fit in the true sense of the word, to really make a difference to your health and well-being, shorter bursts of intense effort are required. In other words, a workout that echoes the training principles of the elite, but is practised in a more convenient and less intimidating format.

Throughout my career, my unwavering belief has been that we can learn a lot from those who push their bodies to extremes. And now science has proven that this is the case, more so than ever as you hit your middle years. Much of what you will read in these pages is evidence gleaned from world leaders in exercise science and anti-ageing research, some of it diluted for our age group, some of it not. It is not something to be feared and will be easier to adopt than you ever thought possible. But the results will astound you. Have you ever seen an athlete with a fat butt? Thought not. I rest my case.

Sarah's background

It's fair to say my adult life has been consumed with food. I am a registered dietitian and nutritionist with a degree in nutrition and dietetics from the University of Surrey, and a PhD in Nutrition and an Accreditation in Sports Dietetics. Since graduating, I have spent much of my career advising people about what they should be eating, many of them fixated with what their bodies can achieve.

I joined Norwich City FC as the team dietitian where Rob Green, an England goalkeeper, and Craig Bellamy, the Wales striker, were among my charges. Subsequently I worked with jockeys and with Kevin Mitchell, the lightweight boxer. Over the years, I have worked as a nutrition adviser to several Premiership football clubs including the teams at Tottenham Hotspur, helping them to achieve the ultimate nutritional status via intricacies such as pinpointing biochemical imbalances in a players' blood samples.

It's certainly been an eye-opener to see how these elite sportspeople dedicate themselves to achieving their best. They are exceptionally disciplined about their diets.

There were no negotiations – no 'I don't like brown rice or courgettes', they just wanted me to tell them what to eat. Nutrition is rife with complexities at that level and I have learned an awful lot about what works and what doesn't through top level sportspeople, but for ordinary mortals the science of staying in shape can be boiled down to pretty simple advice.

What complicates matters is that the rules to which we adhere are often wrong. It has become an overriding passion of mine to set the record straight, to dispel the many myths that circulate about nutrition through my contributions to articles in newspapers and magazines including the *Daily Mail, Top Santé, Reveal* and *Glamour* as well as on shows including *This Morning, Watchdog* and on BBC Radio.

It's satisfying to bust a diet myth if it helps people live simpler and healthier lives and, in the case of this book, to achieve an Ageless Body in the process: skipping meals here and there doesn't matter, I do it myself. In a 24-hour period, it doesn't matter when you take your calories in; whether it's at breakfast, lunch or dinner is irrelevant compared to the overall amount of food we consume. And it's the culmination of this knowledge that I bring to the table. By applying it to my own life, I have gained the Ageless Body I was after, now it's your turn.

'I absolutely get more comfortable in my body and my skin as I get older, more than when I was in my twenties. I think men are intimidated by any woman who's sexually confident, no matter her age.'

Jennifer Aniston

THE AGELESS BODY PROMISE

It's simple: Both Sarah and I have too many time constraints to be bothered with overly complicated diet and exercise plans and have made the assumption (given that you have bought the book and are of a similar age range) that you feel the same. Knowing how flat out most of us are, most of the time, we have made the rules as straightforward and flexible as we can.

Forget calories: Our plans are carefully structured to ensure you are getting everything you need which, incidentally, is significantly less than the 2,000 calories a day officially recommended for women in their forties and fifties. Most days you will be consuming 400–600 calories less than that. You don't have to waste time counting them as we've got that job covered.

Nothing is banned: Well, other than the obvious. Clearly, we don't recommend sweet, fizzy drinks, too much alcohol, or processed and refined foods. But neither are you required to favour one food group over another, nor to shun sugar completely (we cleverly incorporate fruit into many of our savoury dishes to satisfy the sweeter palate and reap the benefits of the nutrients and fibre it provides).

You can skip breakfast: Forget everything you've been told about it being the most important meal of the day, about it kick-starting your metabolism. None of this has been scientifically proven and most of the studies that back breakfast as being essential have rather dubious connections with cereal manufacturers and the like. It's essential for young children, but not adults. If you've felt guilt about having just a black coffee on the run, you can congratulate yourself for taking an important health step. We are both ardent breakfast skippers and proud of it.

You won't starve: Despite the fact you will be 'fasting' for several hours a day, the food avoidance is carefully planned so that you eat when you need to. You will experience hunger, but in a good way. And you will quickly learn that our bodies benefit from it; we are not designed to be drip-fed with snacks throughout the day.

You will come to love exercise: Even if you've loathed the gym for years, you will experience rapid improvements with our workout plans. And the beauty of them is they can be done at home with minimum investment in equipment and no monthly subscription to pay. Plus they're over quickly. Really, what more could you ask?

Weight will fall off: But in a good way. You won't look scrawny (the scourge of the middle age dieter) and drawn. Stick to our guidelines and most of you will drop a dress size in the course of the four-week plan. Once you've reached your desired weight, it's easy to keep off with our maintenance plan and follow-on exercise programmes.

You will live better, for longer: This is more than a diet, it is a lifestyle change for the better. Reams of evidence support our approach in offsetting the risk of diseases and illnesses that begin to strike in the middle years. We can't guarantee you'll live forever, but you will be doing the best you can to expand longevity.

There you have it, some pretty dramatic claims. In the next chapter Peta looks at what happens to the ageing body if you do nothing to slow down the process, and what changes we can expect as the years tick by.

PART ONE

CHAPTER ONE

INTRODUCTION

'I'm almost 50, so I obviously don't have the same body that I had when I was 20. But I also don't have the same mindset either, when I was wracked with self-consciousness and insecurity. Now I really appreciate my maturity as a woman, my depth of spirit and soul and my understanding of who I am and what's important to me.'

Elle Macpherson

EEK – WHAT'S GOING ON?

Whether you have reached this point yet or not, the chances are – since you have purchased this book we can assume you are in the 35–60 age bracket – that you will. One of the most perplexing things about age is that it creeps up and then hits you, bang, completely unawares.

You think you have prepared yourself for the onslaught by accepting the odd crow's foot here, and bulge there. However, few women we have spoken to in the course of writing this book have not experienced a moment of realization, a glance in the mirror, a particularly unflattering photograph, that catapults them into acknowledging that they are no longer in the flush of youth.

There's no telling when or how this will hit. My alarm bells rang when I was slapping on body cream after a shower. There I was, blithely unaware of the impending shock that was to come when I reached my arms. As I flexed them, I noticed the skin on the inside of my elbow creased not in the neatly defined fold it had once formed, but in a crepey fashion that resembled a crumpled bit of tissue paper. Wham. It was a sharp intake of breath moment, the like of which I've heard others talk about.

Interestingly, some months later I was reading an interview with the delectable Gillian Anderson, the *X-Files* actress who has spent the same number of years on this planet as myself. In it, she spoke about her own lightbulb moment, the point at which she realized the years were kicking in. And it was catching sight of her forearms that triggered the reaction. 'I was so shocked that for a few seconds I convinced myself I'd eaten something I was allergic to,' Anderson said. 'We think we're invincible in some way, that age isn't going to touch us, so your response when you see the skin on your hands and your forearms changing is, "Ooh, aah, what the…?"'.

Other friends have spoken about the appearance of jowls or eye bags, a sudden proliferation of age spots or (another of mine) a difficulty applying eye shadow that brings home the fact that eyelids are irreversibly (unless you opt for surgical reversal) drooping. What's crucial, I have found, is to remain in the present, to aim to be as good as you can be now rather than mourning the passing of what cannot be changed. As Anderson said: 'I try and remember in 10 or 20 years I'll be looking back at pictures and my forearms will not have got any better. So appreciate everything you have now.'

There are some aspects of ageing (the crepey infolds, for example) that we cannot halt or reverse without taking extreme measures. Neither should we feel the need to. One of the most satisfying parts of getting older is the self-assurance that it can bring. More confidence, and less worrying about what others think, are the overwhelmingly positive aspects of advancing years. What we focus on in this book are the ageing signs that benefit, not just cosmetically but holistically, from slowing the tide of time.

We all differ in the rate and ferocity with which we age (much more of which later). Some people sail through the middle years without so much as a pound gained or more than an occasional wrinkle making it to their brow. But just in case you have, thus far, avoided the more obvious signs that age is creeping up on you, here is what might be in store and, encouragingly, what we'll be helping to keep at bay with the advice that comes later:

Back fat: My back was always one of my best features, so my friends told me. Too bad I couldn't see it in all its glory for myself, but the glimpses I did get in the mirror did indeed reveal it to be surprisingly toned and muscular. Remarkable, given that it got no special attention. But I turned 40 and it was as if someone had injected adipose cells beneath my bra. Suddenly there were back bulges that had never been apparent before. It is, of course, linked to hormone disruption. Some experts suggest bra fat is a result of thyroid hormones being thrown off kilter, although that's not been proven. More likely it is just another side effect of the body's recalibration as it responds to the ebb and flow of hormones by dumping fat wherever seems most convenient. It's yet another reason why a professional bra fitting (see Boobs) is essential post-35. Going up a circumference size (that's the number of your bra size, the letter being the cup) can lessen the bulging but, in truth, it's the right bra that really makes a difference.

Knees: Looked at your knees lately? Prepare to be unpleasantly surprised. There are two things that might have happened: they get fat or they get wrinkled (dubbed 'kninkles' or knee wrinkles). Catherine Zeta-Jones, Sharon Stone and Gwyneth Paltrow are among the otherwise glamorous women who have fallen prey to the crinkling of their knee joint. What causes it? We need some surplus skin around the knees in order for them to bend. Fine when we are younger, but as we age the collagen beneath the skin's surface breaks down, which causes sagging. The thinner you are, the worse it can look – with less fat plumping out the area above the knee, the effects of gravity appear even greater. On the other hand, older knees can also accumulate fat, becoming puffy and lumpy. They are unlikely to remain your best feature (if they ever were) and we might be thankful that ours is not an age for which miniskirts were designed. However, exercise can help to re-shape your knees or at least the muscles above them, as can moisturizing and generally tending to them as you would your hands.

One piece of good news is that knees needn't necessarily end up beaten, even if you have spent the last decade or two running marathons. Mine are in perfect shape despite my having run most days since I was 11. In 2013, a large study of almost 75,000 runners published in the journal *Medicine and Science in Sports and Exercise* showed that, provided they had healthy knees to start with, runners were at no greater risk of developing arthritis in the joint, even if they jogged into their forties, fifties and beyond.

In fact, most runners had less overall risk of developing arthritis than their non-running counterparts. Even first-time runners, widely believed to be more prone to injuries, are no more likely to suffer knee damage than long-term runners, reported researchers from Germany's Freiburg University Hospital last year. Looking at a group of beginners, average age 40, preparing for their first marathon, the team found that their knees remained essentially unchanged by the training involved with minimal cartilage damage.

Cankles: Age brings many things, but among the least expected is oversized ankles that fuse unapologetically with your calf, hence the term 'cankle'. It has cursed everyone from Hillary Clinton to Patsy Kensit, who do their best to disguise this lower limb widening. Fluid retention can cause blood to pool in the ankles, so it's worth getting checked if they seem more puffy than fat, but otherwise the likely cause is gravity pulling fat stores down toward the ankle and calf area. Working your calf muscles is one way to minimize the appearance of ankle widening.

Belly fat: Call it what you will: muffin top, tummy fat or menopot is the number one gripe among women of a certain age, myself included. I have friends who are well into their forties and fifties who could still wear their size 6 or 8 jeans if it wasn't for the fat spilling over their waistband. It's hormonal (of course). When scientists reviewed decades of research for the International Menopause Society, they concluded that the hormonal shifts of menopause change the distribution of body fat, making it more likely to accumulate in the tummy [3]. When oestrogen levels drop, body fat storage switches from the hips, thighs and buttocks (where it used to be deposited as a fuel reserve for breastfeeding) to the abdomen.

The drawbacks of this are more than just cosmetic: an accumulation of an extra 2–5 inches (5–12.7cm) around the middle can also increase the risk of insulin resistance and cardiovascular disease. Study after study also shows that stress makes abdominal fat worse – even in people who are otherwise thin. Researchers at Yale University, for example, found slender women who had high levels of the stress hormone cortisol also had more abdominal fat [4]. Bad news: it's harder to shift than it was in your twenties; good news: it can be done and we will show you how.

Boob droopage: No other body part is affected by the force of gravity quite as much as the boobs. It's an uphill battle to defy the downward pull, especially when age and breastfeeding do little but accelerate the loss of volume and pertness. It even has a medical name – ptosis. And to find your breasts have dropped to somewhere near waist level is never going to be the most uplifting discovery. You may also find that your breasts change shape, become lumpy or uneven in size. It is fair to say you are entering an age of boob purgatory.

A mixture of gravity and hormones are to blame. As you move beyond your childbearing years, levels of oestrogen and progesterone, the hormones that stimulate the ducts that form the breastmilk delivery system, close up shop. This hormonal flux shrinks down the fat and fibrous tissues that make up the breasts and a part of their support system is lost. Most women find their boobs get smaller as they approach the menopause, but others find that they become a more hefty load.

Scientists at the University of California have proven that boobs age faster than the rest of the body [5]. They developed an algorithm that identified the age of body tissues. Analysing healthy breast tissue from a group of women with an average age of 46, they found it to be, on average, two to three years older than the women's actual age whereas heart tissue, for example, was typically nine years younger than true age. Why? The researchers suspect it's because breast tissue is constantly exposed to hormones. Unfortunately, nothing can reverse the drooping, although target exercise can help to rebuild the support system that makes breasts appear more pert. Again, a professionally fitted bra is essential and can hoist up where Mother Nature falls down.

Flat butt: Some women gain weight in their butt as they age, but the most common complaint is the flattening of a backside. Genes play a role in defining the basic shape of your posterior, as does the natural curve of your back, which can help to create the illusion that your butt is lifted. Likewise, your pelvic tilt determines how wide or narrow your butt appears. But hormonal changes are the biggest determinant as the fat that is stored in your buttocks during your younger years is suctioned away to be deposited on the stomach. Suddenly there's nothing to fill your trousers and you are faced with flat rump syndrome. It's one area that can be improved quite significantly with exercise. Building up the three muscle groups in your behind – the *gluteus maximus, minimus* and *medius* – can add considerable shape and tone. Uphill walking, lunges and squats are perfect butt-boosting exercises as are short bursts of speed. Whoever saw a sprinter with a saggy butt? Precisely.

Bingo wings: I have periods of diligence with my arms, but when I fall off the wagon for a couple of weeks, their demise is shocking. My upper arms can descend from reasonably toned – enough to wear a sundress, at least – to flappy and puffy in as little as a fortnight. The long and short of it is that these limbs require constant attention as the years speed by. The minute you ease up on the dumbbells and tricep dips, your arms will give the game away. Age combined with too little exercise causes the underarm skin to lose its elasticity, fat to accumulate and the dreaded bingo wings to make an appearance. It's no surprise that three-quarters of women in one survey said they disliked their upper arms [6], and another study found that 56 per cent would trade in all their designer shoes to have perfect arms [7]. I'm with you, ladies.

Men are not immune: It's worth mentioning here that, while we women seem to get the raw deal, men are most certainly not immune to the tyranny of ageing. For the over-40 male the cursed trio comprises the moob, the paunch and the love handle. All are the result of body fat deposits and fluid retention, creeping on as metabolism slows and exercise levels drop sharply with age.

Less testosterone (the male sex hormone) combined with increasing alcohol consumption (bad, bad, bad according to every personal trainer we spoke to) often means higher levels of body fat that lead to the development of moobs along with a thicker waistline. As men enter their forties, they start to lose muscle mass more quickly. Given that muscle burns a relatively large percentage of the calories consumed, this means the body gradually loses its ability to burn calories to the max. It's a vicious cycle. Falling hormone levels also leave men fatigued and less inclined to feel like exercising. And like women, men experience a slowing in their metabolism and gain weight more easily later in life. It's no easy ride.

HOW DIET AND EXERCISE HELP

First, a brutal truth: There is no way we can defy ageing altogether. Even the term 'anti-ageing' is not one we feel comfortable about using. We prefer to think of it as recalibrating the body, of re-setting its base points so that we don't accumulate all the adverse signs, symptoms and side effects of ageing at top speed. What we can do is slow it down, not so much halt the progress but reduce the miles per hour at which it is motoring. And the most powerful means to achieving this involve no needles or syringes, scalpels or surgeons.

What we advocate is the only scientifically proven formula for putting the brakes on ageing, albeit in a cutting edge package the like of which you are unlikely to have tried before: diet and exercise.

Quite how powerful diet and exercise can be in terms of keeping us young is an area in which scientific interest has exploded in recent years. Among those looking at the potent effects is Mark Tarnopolsky, a professor of paediatrics at McMaster University in Ontario, who has been at the forefront of investigating how physical activity can prevent premature ageing [8]. In studies, Tarnopolsky has demonstrated a clear advantage to exercising regularly. Using laboratory rodents that were specially bred to repair mitochondria less efficiently than healthy rodents so that ageing was accelerated, Tarnopolsky and his team set about trying to find if activity might stem their decline.

Three months into the trial, one group of mice in his labs were given 5 minutes' access to a running wheel three times a week. He set the wheel at an intense pace so that the mice were forced to run hard and kept up this workload for a total of five months. Other mice did nothing. After the eight months was up, the results were little short of astonishing. Whereas the couch potato rodents were frail and close to death, the gym-rats were brimful of health and vitality with glossy coats, sharp minds and powerful muscles.

Other studies have reached a similar conclusion and the evidence points conclusively to activity being essential for staying youthful. We'll look at this in more detail in the chapters that follow. But a healthy diet enhances those age-defying effects. As you will discover in the next few chapters, we do not advocate cutting out one food group for the sake of another. Or, heaven forbid, starving your way into the next decade. Nor are we huge fans of supplements, vitamin drips and other artificial means of obtaining nutrients (do it if you will, but we consider it largely unnecessary if you stick to our advice).

Likewise, no specific foods are proven to be 'anti-ageing', so don't swallow any of that hype. Your green smoothie might well be rammed with vitamins, but they are not heading straight for your face to erase your wrinkles. Sorry to be the bearers of bad news, but nothing that passes your lips has the power to turn back the clock. What diet can do is enable you not only to boost your longevity, but to hold on to youthfulness and all the health (and cosmetic) benefits it brings for a good while longer.

What we have discovered, both through rigorous evaluation of the available science and through self-testing, is that we can afford to eat fewer calories once we hit 40 and that those calories should be nutrient-dense, that is packed with the right kind of vitamins and minerals to be of benefit, not to cause premature wrinkling. Reducing your daily intake of calories has been proven to slow physical and mental decline. We don't subscribe to the theory proposed by some fasting extremists that you should cut out calories completely for lengthy periods (how achingly miserable), nor even to the alternate day fasting approach that has sky-rocketed in popularity in recent years.

By far the best approach in terms of maintaining youth and vitality is the 4-hour fast, cutting back on food by abstaining from snacks between meals so as to allow your digestive system to restore and re-set during the 4-hour breather. Scientists have known for some time that a lower-calorie diet is a recipe for longer life. Rats and mice reared on restricted amounts of food increase their lifespan by up to 40 per cent. At New York University's Langone Medical Centre, a study found calorie-reduced diets stop the normal rise and fall in activity levels of close to 900 different genes linked to ageing and memory formation in the brain [9].

But there are clear signs it can help humans seeking the fountain of youth too. Research by the US National Institute on Aging suggests that mini-fasting episodes also improve brain functioning, help maintain lean muscle mass, improve insulin sensitivity and boost the release of anti-ageing hormones [10].

Others have shown that mimicking long-term fasting in this way could slow down ageing, add years to life, boost the immune system and cut the risk of heart disease and cancer.

A pilot human trial involving a reduced calorie diet on five days a month, that was published in the journal *Cell*, caused a decrease in risk factors and biomarkers for ageing, diabetes, cardiovascular disease and cancer with no major adverse side effects [11]. It also triggered a drop in amounts of the hormone IGF-1, which is needed for us to grow as young humans, but which also accelerates ageing in later years. Levels of biomarkers linked to diabetes and cardiovascular disease, including glucose, belly fat and C-reactive protein, also dropped when humans ate less. But bone and muscle mass didn't suffer from them eating less.

What you won't experience is gnawing hunger. Our 4-hour fast is purposely designed to sustain you while allowing your blood sugar levels and digestive system time to re-align naturally. We are not designed to snack incessantly and the impact of doing so as we get older can be colossal.

A WORD ABOUT SUGAR

There's emerging evidence that too much sugar and too many of the refined foods that tend to come in plastic packaging are linked to fast ageing. Consumption of sweet, fizzy drinks, for example, was shown to boost cell ageing by University of California biochemists [12]. In a study, they found that telomeres – the protective units of DNA that cap the ends of chromosomes in cells – were shorter in the white blood cells of fizzy drink consumers than in others, a telltale sign that they were ageing more quickly. 'Regular consumption of sugar-sweetened sodas might influence disease development, not only by straining the body's metabolic control of sugars, but also through accelerated cellular ageing of tissues,' said Elissa Epel, the professor of psychiatry who led the study.

Although we urge a reduction in the kind of pre-packaged sugar-loaded foods that have been shown to speed up ageing, we also believe that sugar-shunning has been taken to an unhealthy extreme. We all know we are consuming too much and, with the latest World Health Organization report recommending that we get no more than 10 per cent of our daily energy from added sugars, or those found naturally in juices and honey – equating to about 12 teaspoons a day – you find yourself mentally totting up where it all comes from. Yet it's easy to get swept too far along in the tide of anti-sugar sentiment.

For many, fruit, with its high levels of naturally occurring fructose, is now considered an extra we can do without. Almost without realising it, and against your better judgment, you find yourself cutting down. A good thing? The answer is not as straightforward as you might imagine. Fruit is loaded with beneficial compounds other than its inherent sweetness. Robert Lustig, professor of clinical paediatrics at the University of California, San Francisco, and an expert on childhood obesity, is among the most outspoken anti-sugar campaigners and has called for it to be controlled like alcohol and tobacco. But even he thinks fruit is OK. 'It comes with its inherent fibre, and fibre mitigates the negative effects,' he said. 'The way God made it, however much sugar is in a piece of fruit, there's an equal amount of fibre to offset it.'

That's not to say we think it's a good idea to keep a bowl of berries on your desk and nibble on them, paleo-style, all day. An issue for adults is the high GI content of many fruits. Some, myself included, eat them only to feel more hungry shortly afterwards. We include fruit in our diet plans, but cleverly incorporate them into savoury meals rather than suggesting you eat them in between meals (snacks, as you will discover, are a no-no on the Ageless Diet plan). Far better, we believe, to chuck some apple into a cheese and walnut salad, to combine fruit with other healthful food. That way you lower the fruit's GI, so it's more filling, and you still get the healthy benefits.

WHAT'S YOUR FITNESS AGE?

Scientists at the Norwegian University of Science and Technology have developed a simple test by which you can estimate your own 'fitness age', or how effectively your body is performing for its years [13]. Professor Ulrik Wisloff, director of the KG Jebsen Centre of Exercise in Medicine, has described the low-tech calculation as 'the single best predictor of current and future health'.

Evaluating the fitness, weight and health measurements of almost 5,000 study participants between the ages of 20 and 90, Professor Wisloff and his team used the data to come up with an accurate formula to estimate someone's maximal oxygen uptake, or VO_2max, a measure of aerobic fitness or how efficiently the body transports oxygen to the body's cells. Although VO_2max declines with advancing years, the drop can be slowed considerably with regular exercise. And a favourable VO_2max for your age is linked to a host of health benefits, not least better cardiovascular function and less risk of heart disease and health problems linked to obesity.

It also correlates closely with longevity and is a strong indicator of physical youthfulness or ageing. Ultimately, the lower your VO_2max or cardiorespiratory fitness, the greater the risk is of you developing cardiovascular and heart disease. How fit you are is also increasingly thought to be a stronger predictor of general wellness than, say, weight or BMI alone. Adults aged 60-plus with good aerobic fitness lived longer than unfit people of the same age, regardless of how much body fat they were carrying, according to a study conducted by the University of South Carolina [14]. Others have linked physical fitness to lower levels of high cholesterol, raised blood pressure and osteoporosis.

You can complete the test yourself on the university website – you'll need your waist circumference in centimetres or inches, your resting heart rate (see below), details of how often and how intensely you exercise and your age, and hey presto, you are told how old you are in gym years. The Norwegian scientists admit that their calculator is not scientifically exact but they say it provides a useful 'rough estimate of cardiorespiratory fitness'.

In reality the outcome will be for some a wake-up call. A 45-year-old who exercises moderately and has a 36-inch waistband and a resting heart rate of 72 beats per minute would have a fitness age of 55, for instance. For others, it can provide welcome relief that the Grim Reaper is further away than they thought. Researchers came across one 70-year-old subject with a fitness age of 20.

And my own result was something of a welcome surprise. Keying in my details I was informed that my estimated VO_2max is 49 and my 'fitness age' is 21 – infinitely preferable to my chronological age, given that my 47th birthday is looming ominously. The best news is that, with the workouts we advocate in this book, you can reverse the fitness clock. Years can be knocked off if you step up the frequency and intensity of your exercise – you can realistically attain the fitness level of someone who is much younger and the health prospects of someone half your age.

Peta's journey

During the course of writing this book, my dad died and as I sifted through his belongings, something of an emotional rollercoaster in itself, I found a heap of photographs of myself when I was in my mid-twenties. It startled me how pinched and drawn I looked. How thin, undoubtedly, but also how unhappy I was with my appearance.

Memories of the body trauma I felt at the time came flooding back; all the anxiety and uncertainty about how I looked was etched right there in my worried face. I would spend hours a day exercising, often clocking up 50 miles (80km) a week or more in my trainers. I had run competitively since my primary school days, often running twice a day in training. I also had a gym membership and attended yoga two or three times a week. I ate little and was always hungry. Looking back, my body didn't thank me for it.

Fast forward a few decades and pictures tell a different story. I look a little heavier (thankfully) and more toned and, people have commented when I show them those early photographs, almost definitely younger in physique than I did when I was supposed to be in my prime. Granted, the camera has been kind enough not to hone in on my crow's feet and lines (of which there are plenty), my more papery skin and my eye bags. I am a long way from perfect. Nobody is immune to ageing.

But, by and large, even I can see that the years have not dealt their worst. As I head towards 50, I am the same weight I was, pre-children, at 30. My boobs have slipped a little (thanks breastfeeding), but I can still see my hipbones. My stomach has lost its concave hollowness, but is flat and, I think, more toned than it used to be. And my arms are no longer two scrawny limbs hanging from my hungry frame, but have some shape, some tone. Perhaps the biggest difference is that I am content with my lot. I no longer punish myself over imperfections and don't give a hoot about what others think of my shape. I have reached a sort of nirvana, if there is one, in both body acceptance and appearance, and aim to hold on to it for as long as I can.

Outlined in these pages is a clear guide to how I reached this point. It's a result of years spent interviewing the top honchos in the world of exercise and nutrition science, of grilling leading researchers on precisely what it takes to age healthfully and well. In a nutshell, what I've discovered is that, post-40, three things must become a priority: you need to eat less, exercise harder but shorter and ensure your diet is brimful with age-enhancing nutrients. I spend a fraction of the time I used to exercising, but to better effect. And I remain a breakfast skipper, but eat well the rest of the time. I am no longer permanently calorie-deficient and more energetic, less edgy and anxious as a result.

As you will discover for yourself, there's no need for faddy diets, for lengthy fasts, for green smoothies or collagen-boosting supplements. You will need to make changes to the way you live, eat and exercise, but they are adaptations that will leave you feeling better, not worse. What we advocate is based on hard evidence and compelling new science. And, I think, we are living proof that it works.

Sarah's journey

Apart from one particularly indulgent year I spent as a student in Belfast when I veered towards the chubbier end of the spectrum, I have always been slim. And healthy. I am rarely ill, not succumbing to as much as a cold until our entire family was swiped down with an unpreventable bout of the norovirus five years ago. This has been partly helped by my lifelong love of exercise and also, of course, by my career choice. In my twenties and early thirties I ran, swam, did endless gym workouts, took part in half marathons and the London Triathlon several times. My diet has always been varied and wholesome. I've always thought about the foods I eat in terms of what nutrients they provide; but there is nothing I actively avoid for 'health' reasons.

From my mid-thirties onwards, maintaining this status quo became trickier. I gave birth to two boys 18 months apart and that, coupled with the march of time, has been a reality check: suddenly, in my early forties, keeping my weight under control took much more effort. But through self-experimentation and shifts in what I eat and how I exercise, I have reached the point where I am fitter and stronger than I've ever been, I have lots of energy for the kids – we go cycling, orienteering, camping and it doesn't feel like hard work. And the route to how both Peta and I have achieved this is outlined in this book.

For me, it's been a case of re-adjusting my exercise goals to incorporate lots of body weight exercises, high intensity intervals and a variety of exercise that challenges and surprises my body, often taking it completely unawares. Like Peta, I still run because I love it, but no longer focus my weekly activity solely on clocking up endless miles. I have also learned how to be hungry, and how to get through the day without the limitless snacks that are a scourge to the midlife waistline. Don't get me wrong, I am never near that tetchy, anxious starvation mode where

I'd be irritable and snap at my husband or the children, but I now know I can wait, rather than give in to whatever is in the fridge.

As a nutritionist, everyone expects me to be a saint. I eat healthily and mindfully, aware of what I am consuming but not to the point where choices govern my life. And I do break rules. I am a confirmed breakfast skipper and often don't eat until lunchtime. Contrary to all the official advice and opinion, I have discovered, as you will read further into this book, that skipping breakfast does not make me fat, it does not make me snack on unhealthy foods and it does not mean that I don't get enough nutrients. I rarely snack between my meals, and I make fruit a more integral part of meals rather than snacking on it.

It's been a fascinating journey and one that has proved to me that many of the current recommendations, especially in terms of what we should eat, for women of our age group are simply irrelevant or outdated. In challenging the rules, we have been able to re-write them secure in the knowledge that we know what really works when it comes to attaining a healthy, functional body that looks and behaves more youthfully than it should.

In the next chapter Peta will delve into the science of ageing, and what researchers are discovering about why and how we seem to get older at different rates.

CHAPTER TWO

THE SCIENCE OF AGEING

I t's one thing acknowledging the years are passing at speed, it's another trying to make out how and why it's happening. Getting older – its signs and symptoms, its idiosyncracies and its quirks – are enough to baffle anyone. Most of us (myself included) go through life with, at best, a rudimentary understanding of how our bodies work. Until we reach the point where it helps to know more. In this chapter I'll be unearthing some of the cutting edge science about ageing. What does it mean and can we possibly stop it occurring with such breakneck speed?

WHAT IS AGEING?

We are all getting older, but we are ageing at different rates. You only have to look around you to see it happening – among friends and family, at the school reunion or even among A-listers. Some appear to have luck on their side in apparently holding back the years with relative ease, others to have drawn the short straw on the fast track to frailty. All of us know someone who defies the rules. I have friends who have visibly withered after childbirth and others who have seemingly rejuvenated, knocking decades off appearance-wise and looking younger than they did at 20.

Of course, there is no avoiding the march of time completely. From middle age onwards it eventually comes to us all. But the rate of decline in terms of the loss of muscle, memory, libido and hair, along with the smooth plumpness of skin is certainly not uniform. What fascinates scientists along with the rest of us is what makes us age differently. It's accepted that a birthday is a mere reminder of how many years you have notched up so far, that your chronological age can differ wildly from your biological. But is it simply down to genes and a case of choosing our parents carefully at birth, or can we slow this decline through the way we live?

For decades scientists have analysed how longevity can be predicted using various biological measures, from the shortening of one's telomeres, the DNA-protein 'bumpers' that protect the ends of chromosomes thought to be the biological markers of ageing, to methylation, the process by which DNA gradually transforms in different cells and tissues. Many believe a complex series of molecular events inside our cells that enables communication between the nucleus and of the cell and its mitochondria, the energy providing powerhouses, play a significant role in the ferocity with which we age.

It's been shown that as this intra-cellular communication breaks down, so ageing accelerates. As our bodies become less adept at repairing and restoring healthy mitochondria, they gradually die off. It is when this happens, the thinking goes, that our memory starts to decline, our hair thins and greys and we get slower, become less powerful human beings. In other words, we begin to look and feel our age. It's a convincing theory and one that has substantial evidence to support it. But ageing has also been linked to inflammation and oxidative stress, an accumulation of environmental toxins that causes free radical damage to our DNA.

In short, it remains an unsettled area of science. What we know for certain is that decline is inevitable. None of us can live forever. But science is digging more deeply to find out whether or not we can alter the pace with which ageing happens. In other words, is our ageing cycle pre-determined at birth or can we influence it through diet and lifestyle?

NATURE OR NURTURE?

My hunch has always been that how long and healthily we live is largely dependent on our diet and exercise habits over the decades. Genetics must play a considerable role, of course, but simply to observe those around us who have defied ageing logic surely tells a tale. A great aunt of mine did not change much in appearance in all the time I knew her. She died, at 102, having maintained a relatively youthful bloom, the vitality to walk 2 miles (3.2km) every day and having never conceded to a single grey hair. She adhered to rules that she believed were keeping her alive: the daily exercise, eating the fat on meat, an evening tipple and completing the newspaper crossword. But was it nature or nurture that enabled this to happen? Was it her state of mind, her wilful desire to extend her allotted timespan on this planet that kept her sprightly for so long, or was she just born that way?

In a landmark study, researchers from New Zealand, the UK, the US and Israel analysed data from the Dunedin study in New Zealand, which has been following since birth almost 1000 people born in a specific town of New Zealand during 1972–73 [15]. Researchers based at numerous establishments, including Duke University in the US, set 18 parameters such as lung function, kidney tests, cholesterol and the length of telomeres, those protective caps at the end of chromosomes which shorten with age, to assess an individual's biological age. They measured these markers when the volunteers were aged 26, then 32, and finally at the age of 38, aiming to look at how much they changed over time, to produce a 'pace of ageing' figure.

They found that the years had been much kinder to some than others. In a handful of cases, the past decade had taken no obvious toll on their body's biology. Some participants aged slower than one year per year and stayed a youthful 28.

Others were less lucky. Many participants had biological markers that placed them in their fifties, while one 38-year-old, described as an 'extreme case', was deemed to have a biological age of 61 years. In other words, their body had aged three years for every birthday that had passed. Consequences were disturbing. Given tests normally presented to people over 60, the fast agers performed worse in trials of balance and coordination, mental tasks, such as solving unfamiliar problems, and also reported more difficulties with activities like walking up slopes and stairs.

But they also looked older than their chronobiological age. Students asked to look at photos of the study volunteers and guess their ages consistently rated the fast biological agers as looking older than their 38 years. It was apparent, said the researchers, that only 20 per cent of the ageing process can be attributed to genes. The rest, they concluded, is linked to environments and lifestyles. Proof that we can indeed alter ageing by the way we move and eat.

What twins can tell us

Studies carried out on identical twins who, by definition, have the same DNA and who are brought up together by the same parents have been invaluable in identifying whether it's genes alone that propel us towards wrinkles and frailty. In theory, of course, twins should age in tandem, each losing the markers of youthfulness at the same rate. Nature and nurture appear to have dealt them the same hands, after all. Yet it doesn't always happen that way and scientists were intrigued to find out why.

For over two decades, Tim Spector, professor of genetic epidemiology at King's College London and Director of the Department of Twin Research, has led the way in probing what twins, both identical and fraternal, can tell us about getting older [16]. It baffled him and others to find that identical twins who have the same genes, who shared the same womb and usually experience the same upbringing are so noticeably dissimilar in the rate at which they age and fall prone to disease.

With more than 3500 sets of twins on his books, Spector is now armed with invaluable data about everything including the unique genome sequencing – or decoding of their DNA – of many of his subjects. Every year, participating twins are asked to attend day-long assessments in which Spector and his team log measurements from a range of parameters. All have X-rays and body scans to measure, among other things, bone density. Blood samples are taken, lung function measured, and they are asked to complete a range of psychometric tests to determine any cognitive decline (or otherwise).

What Spector's team noticed was that susceptibility to conditions associated with ageing were not entirely genetic. There were differences in the twins' make up that could not be accounted for by their DNA. His work showed that the 'heritability' of your age at death is only about 25 per cent. Likewise, the chance of a twin suffering heart disease if the other one has suffered already is only 30 per cent. So what shaped the differences in people who were essentially cast from the same mould?

After much investigation and theorizing, Spector concluded that it boiled down to changes occurring in the human epigenome, chemical tweaks to the DNA in our cells that can be influenced by environmental changes. Anything can affect it: long term crackpot diets, illness, smoking, drugs, exposure to pollutants and chemicals, or medication. Observations have proven that cells switched on in one twin can be switched off in another, meaning they have less or more chance of getting a disease or ageing swiftly.

It's a complex science, but one that is fast gaining credence. In a small trial, Finnish researchers managed to locate 10 pairs of identical twins in their twenties with fitness habits at the opposite ends of a scale [17]. In each case, one twin was an avid exerciser, the other a sofa surfer who never hit the gym. All of the volunteers were invited to attend the labs of the University of Jyväskylä where measures of endurance capacity, insulin sensitivity and fatness were taken, as well as scans of their brains.

If ageing were completely down to genetics then results would have been almost as identical as the twins themselves. However, the researchers found stark differences within the pairs. In each case, the non-exercising twin fared worse – their endurance fitness was understandably worse, their body fat higher, their insulin control poorer and their brains contained less grey matter and were less able to respond quickly to stimuli. In short, it seemed clear that their sedentary lifestyle had propelled them towards an ageing body and mind more quickly than their genetically identical sibling.

Likewise, Spector's twin findings have continued to provide huge insight into how and why we age. In one particularly telling experiment, he questioned the twins about their health, weight and, crucially, their activity levels. Over the course of a year, the participants had to record how much they moved about each week, rating the effort their activity entailed from a lazy 1 to an athletic 4. They were also asked about their exercise history, whether they had been sporty or slothful teens, for example.

Blood samples were taken from the participating twins and analysed. It was found that the most active twins had the healthiest levels of white blood cells, considered a marker of a robust immune system. The exercisers also had impressively longer telomeres, the caps at the ends of liquorice lace-like DNA strands. Every time a cell divides, telomeres get shorter. When the telomeres get too short, the cell can no longer divide and scientists believe that ageing occurs as more and more cells reach the end of their telomeres and die. Over time it's what causes muscles to weaken, skin to crease, eyesight and hearing to fade and thinking to cloud.

In fact, the length of the twins' telomeres was directly related to the amount and duration of exercise they did. The moderately active, who managed about 100 minutes a week of an activity such as tennis, swimming or running, had telomeres more similar in appearance to those of someone five or six years younger than those who were at the sedentary end of the scale, mustering only about 16 minutes of movement a week.

The more seriously active, who clocked at least 3 hours a week of moderate to vigorous activity, had telomeres that looked about nine years younger than those of the slothful, a finding that carried true even among sets of twins. There were advantages, too, for those who'd been active in their youth but let things slip. Even if they were moving very little as adults, the previously sporty had effectively lengthened their telomeres through their good workout habits years before.

What it means for all of us is simple. As Spector confirms: 'The act of exercising may actually protect the body against the ageing process.' Music to our ears, indeed.

THE HORMONAL FLUX

No book on the trials of ageing for women can be complete without at least a nod towards hormones. How those blighters rule and overturn our lives from puberty onwards. There's decades of PMS, of mood swings and bloating every month. Then just as the child-rearing years are over, it deals another blow in the form of perimenopausal and menopausal hormone explosion. The average age for menopause in the UK is 52, but symptoms of perimenopause – the hormonal lead up to it – strike up to 15 years before.

For some it's a dawning realization: jeans begin to get tighter, dress sizes to creep up with little or no change to your eating or exercise patterns. For others it's more dramatic. Turn 40 and your waistband seems to thicken overnight. Some women we spoke to felt like they were treading water in a bid to keep the extra pounds at bay. Having ramped up the hours put in at the gym, they were still struggling to offset the effects of hormonal warfare.

One of the reasons we sat down to write this book is that so little practical information is available about the hormonal assault experienced by women of our age that we didn't really understand what was happening ourselves. One minute we were able to plank to within a whisker of a six-pack within weeks, the next we could barely see a waist for the muffin top. Things have improved in recent years, if only marginally.

It used to be that women talked about the M-word through gritted teeth, if at all. But recently celebrities like Angelina Jolie, who announced that she was 'now in menopause' at 39, having had preventive surgery to remove her ovaries and fallopian tubes, and that it was 'nothing to be feared', are speaking out, which has helped to break down the taboo. Even so, our experience is that few are prepared for the sudden transformations that begin to occur weight-wise when the menopause takes grasp. So what IS going on?

Your body is doing the best it can to cope with the tidal wave of hormones that come with the perimenopause and its big sister, but it can feel like a losing battle. Up until their mid-thirties, women tend to carry excess fat on their hips and thighs, while it's men who have the belly issue. But during and after menopause, things start to change: many women's fat storage patterns start to resemble those of men. Dropping levels of oestrogen, the main female hormone, cause weight storage to shift from hips and thighs to the belly, the most risky area to hold on to adipose tissue as it is also likely to settle internally around your vital organs. It's not just unsightly. When menopausal women put on more abdominal fat, they dramatically increase their risk for diabetes, heart disease, stroke and even some cancers.

There's evidence that dwindling levels of oestrogen also cause the body to use starches and blood sugars less efficiently, further increasing the laying down of fat where we least want it. Studies on female laboratory animals have shown that those with lower levels of oestrogen tend to consume more calories and simultaneously move less. Experts think it might influence the same habits in women. Researchers have shown that women in their forties and fifties have higher levels of stress due to lack of sleep and worry about menopausal symptoms. That in itself can increase weight as elevated levels of the stress hormone cortisol can lead to weight gain around the middle.

Then there's the slowing of your metabolism that happens naturally as you get older and is exacerbated by the decline of your muscle mass. Most women gain an average of 10lbs (4.5kg) around the time of menopause. But that needn't be the case. Studies have proven time and again that a diet and exercise plan will not only prevent weight creeping on, but also ward off many other unwanted symptoms of the menopausal years, like hot flushes and poor sleep. Being in the thick of the perimenopause, my own experience is that it almost certainly levels out your mood. There are fewer 'wailing banshee' moments, less of the plummeting into darkness that can plague the hormonally bereft.

By far the biggest benefits, though, are to your body. Nowhere was this more clearly demonstrated than in a study published in the journal *Menopause* involving around 17,000 women, none of whom were taking Hormone Replacement Theropy (HRT) [18]. They were assigned to follow either a healthier diet with plenty of fruits, vegetables and whole grains or their regular diet. After a year, those in the healthier eating diet group not only had fewer hot flushes but were three times as likely to have lost weight.

In another trial conducted as part of the Women's Healthy Lifestyle Project by researchers at the University of Pittsburgh, 535 pre-menopausal women were assessed at regular intervals as they went through menopause [19]. The women were divided into two groups, one group assigned the kind of reduced calorie diet we advocate in our plans (in this case about 1,300 calories daily) along with an exercise plan that led to them using an additional 1000 to 1500 calories a week through sweaty effort. The other group made no lifestyle changes. Five years later, the women in the diet and exercise group saw greater reductions in their waistlines, and they were more likely to have remained at or below their baseline weight.

Along with the scientists, what we've come to realize is that although weight gain is common at midlife, it's not a foregone conclusion. It can be avoided. And that is our aim. It takes concerted effort, both in the gym and the kitchen, but the effects are wonderfully worthwhile.

WHY WE WITHER

Of all the women we have spoken to in the course of writing this book, most claimed the most alarming aspect of hitting 40 was the sudden and dramatic loss of muscle tone. Even among the diligently active, the appearance of crepey skin and hanging flesh in place of previously taut definition, the sagging of body parts that had been pert and youthful, was disquieting to say the least. What on earth causes such rapid demise, they wondered.

Around 40 years ago, science uncovered the answer. Major studies revealed that from the mid-thirties onwards, all of us begin to lose muscle mass, a process known as sarcopenia (a Greek word for loss of flesh). It is to muscles what osteoporosis is to bones: a sly, destructive progression that leeches the body of its muscle strength without warning but sometimes with catastrophic effect.

What early studies showed is that from around the third decade of life onwards sarcopenia steals an average one-fifth of a pound of muscle a year. Beyond the age of 50, it adopts an almost parasitic speediness, bleeding the body of up to 1lb (0.45kg) of muscle every 12 months. An 80-year-old who does nothing to stop the rapid decline typically has one-third less muscle mass than a 20-year-old.

Both men and women are affected (men – with their naturally greater muscle mass – experience a sharper decline) but, with few warning signs that it's happening, most of us remain unaware of it until things start to sag and droop. What has concerned experts, particularly those who first identified it, are the effects this incremental loss of strength can have on healthy ageing.

Diminished muscle mass is likely to raise blood lipid levels and body fat, particularly the visceral fat that accumulates around vital organs, which is partly why sarcopenia has been linked to the development of obesity and heart disease. It has also been shown to affect insulin resistance and the onset of Type 2 diabetes; some small studies have shown an association between sarcopenia and mortality from cancer. Lower levels of lean muscle tissue mean that the body's metabolic rate – its ability to burn calories – slows down, and since stronger and thicker muscle tissue helps to keep bones healthy, advanced sarcopenia could also lead to weaker bones and osteoporosis, studies have shown.

A shortfall of the early studies is that they looked, almost exclusively, at sedentary populations, people who rarely moved the muscles that were found to be withering. It led scientists to wonder if a targeted programme of physical activity might in some way help to stem the muscular free fall. Why our muscles wither with age began to carry newfound significance and, in the last decade, a growing number of research bodies have become captivated by the possibility that we can slow down the rate at which our muscles age.

What's crucial, they have discovered, is that working the muscles through any physical activity is helpful. But overloading them with resistance exercise or weight training is by far the best preventative measure. It seems that muscle mass can be improved – sometimes significantly – with this kind of training, even after the onset of sarcopenia, although the earlier you can begin pumping iron and performing the kind of body weight exercises we advocate in Part Two of the book, the better.

How does it work? Resistance exercise triggers tiny tears in myofibrils, the proteins that cause muscles to contract. Cells are activated around the area where this micro-damage occurs and the body recruits protein to repair and strengthen the muscle. In effect, resistance training acts as a catalyst for muscle growth. Research by Robert Wolfe, a professor in geriatrics at the University of Arkansas, suggested that the optimum sarcopenia-busting programme should involve a high intensity of effort (using 70 per cent of the maximum weight someone perceives they can lift) for all major muscle groups [20].

Other researchers have recommended one weekly resistance session for the muscles in the chest and triceps (backs of the arms), one for the back and biceps and one for the legs and shoulders. 'All studies to date show that resistance training is highly important in adult life,' says Avan Aihie Sayer, a professor in geriatric medicine at the University of Southampton. 'The earlier you can start it in adulthood, the better, but it is never too late. You can't stop sarcopenia completely, but you can modify the way you lose muscle which, in turn, may enhance the way you live your life.'

There's no doubt that sarcopenia is being taken more seriously than ever as a threat to healthy ageing. Pharmaceutical companies have established muscle metabolism units specifically to look at drugs that might eventually be used to treat the condition. But a reliance on medication is the last chance saloon; much of the onus remains on us. Our Ageless Body workout plans are designed specifically to combat muscle loss as well as the other physical signs of ageing.

AND WHY WE SHRINK

Some loss of bone strength after the menopause is inevitable. As we get older, the body's ability to replace new bone tissue slows, the bones shrink slightly and become brittle, making them more likely to collapse and break – a condition known as osteoporosis. Known as a silent disease, osteoporosis can take hold without you realising, until a bone breaks in response to a relatively small trip or fall. One in three women will eventually suffer from the condition.

And the closer we get to the menopause, the more dramatic the effects become. As oestrogen, a bone-protective hormone, falls, so the risk of brittle bones rises. Five to seven years after menopause women can lose up to 20 per cent of their skeletal strength. What many women in their mid-thirties onwards don't realize is quite how close they are to that marker, already with a lesser degree of bone loss called osteopenia.

Weakened bones are not only a health risk, they result in an older looking and behaving skeleton. Most of us lose at least one-third of an inch (1cm) in height every decade after the age of 40. By 80, many women will be as much as 3.15 inches (8cm) shorter than they were in their twenties. Those women who shrink in height and hunch over? They almost certainly have osteoporosis. Many women with the condition suffer tiny fractures to their spine without even realizing it, causing a shortening of stature.

But other factors relating to bone health are at play. As we get older, the jelly-like disks between the vertebrae of the spine that act as its shock absorbers start to dry out and get thinner and flatter. The spine becomes permanently compressed. Strength and tone, especially in the abdominal muscles that support the spine and its structure, diminished without the right kind of exercise, can add to your lack of height.

At 5 feet 5 inches (165cm), I really cannot envisage getting any nearer to the ground. So what can we do to keep our skeleton, and our stature, healthy? A healthy diet comprising all of the essential micro- and macronutrients is important, but activity shares that spot at the top of the list. Israeli researchers found that people who engaged in moderately vigorous exercise lost only about half as much height as those who stopped exercising in middle age or never exercised at all [21]. Any weight bearing exercise – that's an activity that requires your body to carry the burden of its own weight like running, walking, skipping or aerobics – is good, whereas non-weight bearing activity – that in which your body is supported in some way, as it is on a bike or in a pool – has minimal effect on bone-building.

Resistance training is also important. We can't stress enough how the body weight circuits and dumbbell exercises you'll read about in Part Two can help to maintain your body on the inside while transforming it (for the better) on the outside. Researchers in Austria have been looking at how beneficial weight training can be in terms of ageing bones. Experts from the MedUni Vienna prescribed weekly buddy-led strength training sessions for older volunteers and early results show that it is particularly beneficial for increasing hand strength, and thus enabling people to live indepen dently [22]. And another trial at the Department of Health Sciences at University of Jyväskylä in Finland found that post-menopausal women, all of whom had mild knee osteoarthritis, asked to do high impact exercises like jumping, squat thrusts and burpees for 12 weeks had improved cartilage and a reduction in the rate of bone loss [23].

But the simplest of exercises can help. When 60 premenopausal women, aged 25 to 50, were asked to jump 10 times as high off the ground as they could manage twice a day with short breaks (30 seconds) between each jump, they significantly increased their hip bone mineral density after four months by 0.5 per cent. If it doesn't sound much, let's put it into perspective: the control group of the same age who didn't jump daily lost 1.3 per cent of their bone density over the same three-month period.

FACE IT

Looking after your bones by packing in vitamin D, plenty of calcium-containing leafy green vegetables and exercising appro- priately can have other age-defying benefits. As we get older, our facial bones including our eye sockets, upper jaw and nose begin to change. Writing in the journal *Plastic and Reconstructive Surgery*, University of Rochester researchers revealed how alterations to bone structure affect the youthfulness of our appearance [23].

For example, as eye sockets get bigger, the angle of the bones beneath the eyebrows decreases. The upshot? Frown lines can form on your forehead and crow's feet at the corner of your eyes. They found that the angle of the jawline increases with age, causing a loss of definition in the lower face and the appearance of the dreaded jowls as well as sagging skin and a crepey neck, it was reported.

Although these changes occurred in both sexes, many occurred earlier in women, often between the ages of 20 and 36. In men, most of the changes occurred between middle age (41 to 64) and old age (65-plus). The outcome of the study will almost certainly be used to develop some new cosmetic facial rejuvenation technique. But it also underlines the importance of maintaining bone structure and health as the Ageless Body plans propose.

Adopt a youthful posture

It's not just our face and skin that display the telltale signs of ageing. With advancing years come noticeable changes to posture, with a youthful stance often being replaced by hunched, rounded shoulders. So, shoulders back, tummy in, stand to order.

Foetal position
Women's bodies often revert to the foetal position as we get older: the head and shoulders shift forwards, the chest curls inwards and the spine crunches into a 'C' position as the pelvis tilts forward.

Tip: Practise standing up straight several times a day with your back to a wall, heels touching the skirting board and with shoulders and back of the head touching the wall.

Duck feet

As the core muscles that support the spine weaken with age, particularly so after the menopause, so balance diminishes. Some of us compensate by turning the feet and toes outwards in a subconscious attempt to widen our support base.

Tip: As well as consciously trying to walk and stand with feet pointing straight ahead, calf raises (lifting up onto the balls of your feet) can help to improve walking style by strengthening muscles in the lower legs, while exercises targeting the back extensors, neck flexors and pelvic muscles can also be helpful.

Dowager's Hump

The one we all dread. A hallmark of old age, the so-called Dowager's Hump, or kyphosis, is characterised by a rounded upper back sometimes with a visible hump. Shoulders are usually hunched forward and hips are rounded inwards. It is caused by partial collapse of the spine due to compression of the vertebrae and is often a result of osteoporosis.

Tip: Any weight bearing exercise will help, but resistance training with bands or weights will strengthen essential bones, ligaments and muscles.

In the next chapter Sarah looks at how diet affects ageing. She will explain the underlying principles behind the Ageless Body eating plans, why and how our bodies need change as we get older, and how we should overhaul what we are currently consuming in order to stay looking (and feeling) our best.

CHAPTER THREE

EATING FOR AN AGELESS BODY

When Peta and I first started chatting about our own approaches to eating, it was remarkable how similar our dietary habits were. And also how far removed many of them were from the recommended advice that we are spoon-fed by health authorities. Neither of us eats breakfast. Peta has her first meal as a brunch at around 11 a.m. whereas I hang on a little longer, preferring an early lunch as my first meal.

We don't snack or graze, the approach that's become popular for maintaining energy levels and keeping the metabolism ticking over, preferring instead to eat satisfying larger meals usually twice, sometimes three times, a day. We eat considerably less than we did in our twenties and barely come close to the 2000 calories a day recommended for women of our age. We sometimes exercise on an empty stomach. We don't avoid those dietary pariahs – carbs, fat and fruit – but incorporate them carefully into our diets.

And yet we don't feel guilty about any of it. Why should we when we are healthy, fit and happy, living proof that our regimen works? We rarely get ill and hardly ever get injured. Our weight barely fluctuates.

We must be doing something right. Indeed, our view is that much of what we are told about when and how much to eat is outdated advice and too generalized, in that it doesn't take into account the specific changes that occur to our bodies as we get older and the steps we need to take in terms of food intake to deal with these.

What's more, science has proven that many of the rules that have governed our dietary thinking until now are flawed. In this chapter, I'll be unravelling some of these myths about food and outlining the eating habits that will help you to achieve your Ageless Body rather than accelerate ageing.

YOU NEED TO EAT LESS AS YOU AGE

One of the unfortunate realities of getting older is that it's much harder to get away with over-eating. Whereas you could get away with weekend binges at 20 or 30, it suddenly seems that every extra morsel that passes your lips seems to find some way of clinging to your frame as you enter the next few decades of life. It's no figment of your imagination either. The truth is you need less energy (or fewer calories) simply to survive at 40 than you did at 30, and the requirement decreases proportionately with the advancing years.

Let's look at why that happens. Energy (provided by calories in the form of food and drink) is needed by the body just to keep everything ticking over, to maintain the physiological equilibrium that is medically referred to as our basal metabolic rate (BMR). BMR is influenced by many factors: lean body mass, age, sex, thyroid hormones and protein turnover so it ebbs and flows at different stages of life. In addition, our bodies use energy to digest and absorb food, to regulate body temperature (known as thermogenesis) and to fuel any exercise or physical activity we fit into our schedules. All of this is accepted as fact. What science is beginning to question is quite how significantly our energy needs change with age.

The World Health Organization has estimated that our BMR decreases by an average 2.9 per cent in men and 2 per cent in women over each decade. At the same time, there are shifts in our body composition as we age: there's a greater proportion of fat to lean muscle mass and pounds creep on here and there with each decade that passes. Ageing also affects the efficiency with which we digest and metabolize food, that's the energy cost of eating or diet-induced thermogenesis (DIT, for short). Results of research tend to show that DIT is higher in younger people than older people, that a 20-year-old would use up more energy eating the same dish of macaroni cheese as a 70-year-old.

So where does that leave us? Official Department of Health recommendations in the UK are that the average woman who is a healthy weight needs to consume 2000 calories a day to stay in energy balance, that is neither gaining nor losing weight. This figure is based on an equation that takes into account assumed physical activity levels (PALs) relative to BMR. With the average PAL for a woman aged between 19 and 50 estimated at 1.5 and her average BMR being 1300 (that is the equivalent to the body using just under 1 calorie a minute during a 24-hour period while at complete rest), advisers multiplied the figures and rounded up to 2000 calories a day.

From our late thirties onwards, neither Peta nor myself has eaten anything near that daily amount. We maintain a healthy weight by eating significantly less. It's no coincidence either. Recent studies of women aged 35–50 have found that both metabolic requirements and PALs are overestimated, so it is highly unlikely the average woman in that age group needs 2000 calories per day. Despite this, official advice is to stick at that level until you hit 51, when the suggestion is to cut your intake to 1900 calories, until age 75 when you can supposedly stay slim on 1810 daily calories.

In our opinion it's still too much. We are certainly not advocates of starvation, but our own experiments have shown that the optimum intake for women of our age and older who want to stay in good shape is some 300–400 calories below the accepted norm. As such, our Ageless Body is based on significantly less than official guidelines dictate. Don't get me wrong, we will ensure you pack in the nutrients, never go hungry and are brimful with health, but weight loss and maintenance will become that much easier.

THE BIG BREAKFAST MYTH

So, here's a thing: Breakfast is not the most important meal of the day for adults. Children need it, but the rest of us can go without and might even benefit from it. Who'd have thought it? After years of being told that to breakfast like a king is essential to fire up the metabolism, that breakfast eaters are slimmer, more quick thinking and more inclined to eat healthily, the weight of evidence has turned. It's now known that while some of us are naturally inclined to be breakfast eaters, others are not. And it makes not a blind bit of difference to our well-being.

Both Peta and myself fall firmly into the category of breakfast skippers. Particularly as we get older, we have found that we simply don't need calories first thing in the day. Peta says missing breakfast, for her, wasn't a conscious decision, but more of a gradual adaptation. As she got older, she ate less because she didn't feel hungry when she first got up and eventually found she was avoiding food altogether until around 11 a.m. when she 'brunches' to see her through to an evening meal. When she does occasionally eat first thing – on holidays or when staying with friends – Peta says she's invariably starving by lunchtime. Without doubt she ends up eating more than usual. It's much the same for me. I eat more sensibly and healthily throughout the day when I've avoided breakfast.

Yet, for both of us it was something of a guilty secret for the last few years. We are both health specialists and, of all people, we each felt we should publicly uphold the belief that eating first thing is good practice. But the inconsistencies were too glaringly obvious and we eventually began to voice our concerns about conventional advice. Fortunately, as we 'came out' as closet breakfast-shunners, so science and popular opinion began to support our claims that breakfast was not strictly necessary.

Papers began to emerge in esteemed publications that questioned whether there are any confirmed and specific health benefits from breakfast-eating first thing. Experts writing in the *American Journal of Clinical Nutrition*, for example, suggested that only a handful of rigorous trials had ever really put breakfast-eating to the test and most conclude that whether you skip it or not, it has little effect on weight gain [25]. It only compounds the scepticism I've long felt about the studies that recommend we should be packing in the calories first thing and which, on closer inspection, are often funded by cereal or breakfast bar companies. In a full circular swing, many have jumped on board with us in thinking that breakfast is overrated and that, as we enter our forties, our waistlines benefit more if we go without.

Indeed, over the last couple of years we've noticed a huge shift in opinion about our particular dietary vice. It no longer has to be a secretive habit. Everyone is at it. From the most glamorous

40-something mummies at the school gates to ageless celebrities, it has become something of a badge of honour to have completed the morning school run or a pre-work gym session without so much as a morsel having passed your lips. The uber-glamorous Joanna Lumley has said 'I quite often don't have breakfast', her theory being that eating early in the day kick-starts her body into wanting more and more food. 'I find it helps not to wake my stomach up because if I have a big breakfast I'd be ready for a snack at 11 a.m. and then a three-course lunch, then I'd be ready for tea and a cocktail and then an enormous dinner,' the actress has said. Another who has championed breakfast avoidance is the ever-lithe Liz Hurley who has said that she maintains her figure by consuming only mugs of hot water and an occasional espresso in the morning, and that 'the only meal I have is dinner'.

Some scientists have backed the concept that skipping breakfast can mean fewer calories consumed, not more. German researchers looked at the food intake of 280 obese adults and 100 adults of normal weight. Subjects were asked to keep records of everything they ate over two weeks. For both groups, a large breakfast simply added to the total number of daily calories they consumed. Whether they ate a large breakfast or none at all did not affect their remaining calorie intake throughout the day. In other words, you don't always compensate for a hearty breakfast by eating less throughout the day. At Cornell University, several studies have added weight to the argument that depriving people of breakfast is not necessarily a bad thing. It can help you lose weight – not gain it.

In general, the consensus is now that we can miss the morning meal without worrying about putting on weight. This was shown by a team from the University of Alabama who recruited nearly 300 volunteers, all of whom wanted to lose weight [26]. The researchers randomly assigned each of the subjects to follow one of three sets of dietary rules: stick to their current eating habits, cut out breakfast or eat an early morning meal every day. After four months, the subjects returned to the Alabama labs to be weighed. Nobody had lost much weight, but the breakfast eaters fared no better on the scales than those who had skipped it, putting to bed the idea that a morning meal somehow 'kick-starts' the metabolism.

Dr James Betts, a researcher in nutrition and metabolism at the University of Bath, also carried out a breakfast study [27]. He allocated a group of lean subjects to either a 'fasting' group or a 'breakfast' group for six weeks. Rules were simple: the fasting group were to consume no calories until 12 p.m. each day, with the breakfast group eating 700 calories before 11 a.m. – 350 within two hours of waking up. Measurements of their blood sugar, cholesterol levels and resting metabolic rates were taken and the volunteers were issued with an activity-tracking device.

At the end of the trial, the breakfast eaters had experienced no improvements in snacking frequency or portion sizes or any change in their resting metabolism, contrary to popular opinion. There was one significant advantage from the morning meal – people who ate it moved around more, burning an extra 442 calories as a result. Fasters were more sluggish first thing. 'The main finding from our study is that people who eat breakfast burn more calories,' Dr Betts said. 'Most people would think this is because of reduced snacking and increased metabolic rate but actually this is due to moving around.' Of course, those who had eaten breakfast had consumed more calories to start with, meaning the benefits of the activity in terms of weight loss were effectively offset.

This emerging evidence paves the way for a deeper look into how meal timings work for our bodies. There's much more to be learned about if or how breakfast affects mood and concentration levels or whether the perception of having low levels of energy might mean some people are less inclined to be active. As with many things diet-related, there can be no hard and fast rules. We are all different and it's a matter of finding out what works for you.

What we know for certain is that skipping breakfast won't make or break diet success. In our view (and the view of an increasing number of nutrition experts) breakfast is just another meal. It contains calories and eating these calories will impact on your weight in the same way that eating at any other time of day will. Consuming food first thing will help you to shed pounds only if you eat less (or move more) overall throughout your remaining waking hours to compensate for the extra calories you've had in your morning croissant, coffee or scrambled egg. Latest data suggests this is rarely the case. So, eat breakfast if you really feel the need, but don't fret about skipping it if you don't.

WHAT ABOUT FITNESS-FASTING?

Another long-held myth is that you should never exercise on an empty stomach. Well, both Peta and I have long flouted that rule, too. Both of us have been known to set out for the occasional (once or twice a week maybe) early morning workout with no pre-fuelling. Again, scientific evidence has now confirmed that we are not completely bonkers and that what we've practised for years is not dangerous. In fact, what has become known as the 'fitness-fast' might even be of benefit when it comes to warding off that middle-aged waistline.

Celebrities love it. Tracy Anderson, the fitness guru who guides the likes of Gwyneth Paltrow, Jennifer Aniston and Christie Turlington, speaks about it in glowing terms. And when Peta interviewed Madonna's personal trainer, Nicole Winhoffer, she said the perfect start to the day is some form of cardio exercise performed on an empty stomach. 'I do it every morning,' Winhoffer said. 'I believe it has to be slow – your heart rate shouldn't rise above 128bpm – but it will pull energy directly from your fat stores.'

So how exactly does it work? With the body forced into a fasting state during sleep, it is primed for optimal fat-burning when we first wake up. Because carbohydrate stores are depleted overnight, a pre-breakfast workout will force the body to tap into its energy reserves, burning off calories stored as fat instead. It's an approach that has been popular among body builders and weight lifters for years and some studies, including one at Kansas State University, have shown that a kilogram of fat is burned off sooner during morning exercise carried out after an overnight fast than when doing the same exercise in the afternoon [28].

According to Mike Gleeson, a professor in exercise biochemistry at Loughborough University, fitness-fasting isn't just a fad, but based on scientific reasoning. 'Food releases insulin, a hormone that blunts fat-burning, into the bloodstream,' Professor Gleeson told us. 'Insulin levels are at their lowest of the day when you first wake up which does mean that pre-breakfast is the optimal time for fat to be burnt.' Most people practise fitness-fasting prior to cardio-vascular activities like running or cycling, but Gleeson says that in order to activate the mechanisms that burn fat and tone muscle, it's a good idea to include some resistance or weight training in your fasted workouts.

We've certainly found a couple of fitness-fasts a week works for us, but are also aware that they won't suit everyone. If you are an avid breakfast eater, for example, you might not feel the same urge to head out on an empty stomach. A study published in the journal *Medicine and Science in Sports and Exercise* several years ago appears to prove this point. Researchers asked a group of exercisers to ride on indoor bikes one morning after eating a small breakfast and another morning after eating nothing at all. On an empty stomach, the subjects simply got tired more quickly and stopped pedalling 30 minutes sooner than those who had eaten.

The theories of exercise science don't translate into practice for everyone and some researchers have suggested that some people also over-compensate by guzzling more calories when they finish. However, if like Peta and myself, you find it helps your enthusiasm for getting out in the morning as well as your fat burn and appetite control, then don't feel guilty about trying it. We'd suggest no more than a couple of sessions a week of fitness-fasting and stick to shorter sessions to start with, but give it a try.

GENERATION GRAZE

Grazing, as we've come to refer to snacking, first became really popular in the 1990s when studies suggested that eating little and often was best for the body. It's a theory that stemmed from science surrounding what is known as the thermic effect of food – the calories burned in order to break down and metabolize the food we eat. In the past, we were encouraged to take advantage of this process by eating little and often. The idea was that we could stoke up our metabolic rate and gain a net advantage of energy used up.

Large meals, we were told, serve only to burden the digestive system, causing bloating and lowered energy as the body struggles to process them.

Eating the traditional three square meals a day would cause a sluggish metabolism, slow down the rate at which we could shed surplus pounds and lead to hours when, without food, our blood sugar and energy levels would drop. Without snacks, we were led to believe everything would suffer: our attention span, our workouts, our waistlines.

As a result, we became snack-obsessed, the food industry fuelling our desire to eat on the run with endless new mini meal-sized, pre-packaged products in supermarkets, coffee shops and juice bars. People carry around small pots of mixed seeds, edamame beans or sriracha peas alongside bags of almonds, cashews or dried mango chunks. These are not just nibbles for boredom avoidance and a supply of healthy nutrients. They are billed as survival fuel, essential for firing up energy levels, preventing blood sugar from dipping to a debilitating low and, of course, for avoiding temptation when it comes to the biscuit tin.

Grazing is now so embedded in our lifestyles. It's big business for the food industry, which has a conveyor belt of tempting new products to ensure we keep eating. Manufacturers have perpetuated the myth that hunger is a bad thing and that we constantly need food at our fingertips. Employers striving to keep staff happy and productive now offer free snacks in the workplace, granola bars and smoothies increasingly provided on tap in office kitchenettes. High-flying executives are put through 'energy for performance' courses on which they are encouraged to drip-feed their brainpower throughout the day with regular nibbles. Snacks are recommended by personal trainers to boost exercise performance and recovery and by many nutritionists to avoid weight gain.

Yet we believe the craze to graze that marked a move towards incessant eating has not only contributed towards the obesity epidemic but also makes it incredibly difficult to keep weight at bay after 40. We're not the only ones who think this way as, scientifically, snacking is falling out of favour. Science has now proven that, rather than small meals boosting the thermic effect of food and consequent calorie burning, the reverse is true. One study investigated the effect of eating the same food as one large meal or three small snacks and found the thermic response to the large meal was 66 calories higher than the total of the three snacks. It can be argued that over time this 66 calories could be significant in helping to manage weight.

Repeated studies have shown that a larger meal eaten in one go uses up calories more efficiently than if the same foods were eaten as a sequence of snacks. In other words, you'll retain more of the calories eaten as snacks than you would had you eaten the food as one meal. And the chances are they'll head straight to your middle or hips.

There are other unhealthy side effects that take on more significance as the years roll on. Take a group of researchers from the Netherlands who reported in the journal *Hepatology* that, compared with three large meals a day, frequent snacks were more likely to cause cholesterol stores in the liver to rise along with the accumulation of harmful fat around the waist. Dr Mireille Serlie, who led the trial at the Academic Medical Centre in Amsterdam, said her findings clearly suggested 'that [...] by cutting down on snacking' and encouraging less frequent meals each day 'over the long term may reduce the prevalence of non-fatty liver disease' [29].

Meanwhile, findings by Czech Republic scientists suggested that two hearty meals a day achieved far better blood sugar control for people with Type 2 diabetes than constant nibbling on six daily mini meals [30]. All volunteers in the 12-week study lost weight. Yet the findings, published in *Diabetoligia*, showed that participants eating twice a day lost around 7lbs (3.7kg), compared with just over 3.5lbs (2.3kg) for the snackers.

If you are serious about an ageless body, then our recommendation is not to 'eat on the go', to keep snacking to a bare minimum and to re-align your meal timings to an approach that complements your body, not wages a war against it. As you will see in the next section, it's perfectly normal, and healthy, to go hungry.

THE 4-HOUR FAST – HOW IT WORKS

All of this brings us to one of the most important premises of our Ageless Body Diet Plan: the 4-Hour Fast. Don't let that name put you off. In essence, we are advocating eating only when you are hungry (and we mean really hungry, not bored), when you have a physical need for food. For most people, this naturally occurs around every 4-hour mark throughout the day, but for some of you it may be a slightly shorter or longer duration. The rules are simple: after you have eaten, you then fast for another 3–4 hours.

If you are a grazer, it can take some getting used to. But within a few weeks of recalibrating your hunger cycle, you will never look back. Stretching out the kind of daily fasting periods we naturally practise at night has been shown to override some of the adverse health effects of unhealthy eating and help to prevent diabetes, liver disease and, crucially for readers of this book, middle-aged weight gain.

Let's look at why this works. Our livers, intestines, muscles and other organs are designed to operate at peak efficiency at certain times, but to need rest at others. This downtime is critical for processes like cholesterol breakdown and glucose production to take place. Grazing throughout the day throws this metabolic cycle off kilter and results in a cascade of hormonal disruption.

When we eat, particularly food rich in carbohydrate, our blood glucose levels rise and our pancreas starts to release the hormone insulin in a bid to control them. Glucose is the main fuel that our cells use for energy, but it is important that high levels are not left circulating in the blood as it increases the risk of diabetes. Insulin's job is as a regulator, keeping these blood sugar levels neither too high or too low by removing it from the blood and putting it into the cells of the muscles and liver where it is stored in a stable form to be used as and when needed. It's a role it does well unless the pancreas becomes overloaded due to frequent demands for its control.

But insulin also has a role in the metabolism of fat. It inhibits a process known as lipolysis, the release of stored fat from body fat cells into the blood to be used as energy. At the same time it moves fat from the blood into other cells to be stored. What this means is that a constant release of insulin in the body leads to increased fat storage and its doppelgänger – weight gain. This is ultimately where our craze to graze falls down. Constantly eating lots of sugary and carbohydrate-rich food and drink triggers the release of more and more insulin to deal with the constant surge of glucose into our bloodstreams.

Your pancreas copes all right to begin with, pumping out larger quantities of insulin and depositing fat around the body's cells. But eventually it becomes overwhelmed. Cells become resistant to the large amounts of insulin being produced and your body enters a pre-diabetic state known as metabolic syndrome. It's not good news. Not only does it increase the risk of heart disease, stroke and cancer it also interferes with normal hormone balance and can affect your mood, appetite and sense of vitality and well-being.

Our two-pronged approach to this is simple: we advocate 1) cutting back on carbohydrates and replacing them with more vegetables and healthy fats, and 2) a 4-hour fast between meals, not drinking or eating anything but herbal tea, water or black coffee.

The benefits of the 4-hour fast are both immediate and long lasting. After around 2 hours of eating, the body begins to enter what those in the medical world call 'the fasted state'. Blood glucose level begins to drop, insulin secretions slow down and there's a rise in a different hormone called glucagon. Just as insulin signals the fed state, glucagon signals the fasted state and it has opposing – and far more appealing – actions. It breaks down and mobilizes stores of carbohydrate and fat, and also inhibits lipogenesis (or fat storage). The first few times you stick to the regimen you might find yourself feeling hungry or low on energy, but that won't last long. Your body is a super-efficient machine and will re-set itself to this new approach to meal timings. So if you can distract yourself from these feelings for 20 minutes or so, you will find that they pass and there is no need to snack. Before long it will become second nature. You'll find yourself passing coffee bars and 24-hour food shops with a certain smugness that comes with knowing you've broken the snacking cycle.

Plus, it's worth hanging in there. After 3–4 hours without eating, there are significant improvements in weight control and appetite regulation, but also in holding back the years. These mini fasts between meals limit the action of an age accelerating hormone known as Insulin-Like Growth Factor 1 (IGF-1). This hormone has growth-promoting effects on almost every cell in the body and high levels of IGF-1 are associated not only with speedy ageing but an increased risk of cancer. A 4-hour fast has been shown to reduce the amount of IGF-1 your body produces as well as switching on a number of repair genes to prevent damage to your DNA.

By training yourself to wait for the next meal your body will soon get used to leaving space between meals and it'll become a walk in the park. Plus the recipes and food plans we've provided in Part Two of the book are not only delicious, but filling and satisfying too, which makes sticking to it a whole lot easier.

In summary, here's what our 4-hour fast will help you to achieve:

- Weight loss
- Improved body composition – fewer bulges
- Lower levels of IGF-1, the ageing hormone
- A rested pancreas and improved insulin sensitivity
- Better balanced hormones – and a better mood
- A younger looking and feeling body

BALANCE YOUR MACRO- AND MICRONUTRIENTS

It's not only advice about how much we need to eat that we think is outdated; current recommendations about the macro- and micronutrients we need to stay healthy are also, in our opinion, no longer relevant to our lifestyles, particularly as we get older. There are so many flaws to the eatwell plate, a UK government policy tool that is used as the standard means of suggesting how different foods should contribute towards a healthy balanced diet, that it would be unreasonable to list them all here. For one, healthy fats are much maligned and grouped together with unhealthy fats and sugary drinks like cola as foodstuffs to be limited.

But one of the eatwell plate's biggest downfalls is that it recommends we base all our meals on starchy carbs, telling us to include bread, potatoes, rice or pasta at every meal so that they constitute one-third of our daily calories. It is advice based largely on the energy needs of generations who lived in a previous century. Our carbohydrate needs today are considerably less because our lives are so much more sedentary. Who needs a big bowl of starchy cereal just to sit at a desk all morning? Given the latest evidence, this carb-loading approach is far from sound advice for weight loss, particularly for our age group.

In our eating plan, we suggest only one meal a day based on healthy carbs. We certainly don't want you to severely restrict carbs or eliminate them altogether. But a large amount of carbohydrate delivered into the bloodstream means body tissues use it as a fuel instead of the circulating fats, so the fats get stored where we least want them. For example, if you have a slice of bread and butter, the bread gets metabolized first so the butter is laid down as fat. If you just had the butter, your body would metabolize that first.

Our aim is to mobilize your fat stores. This can't be done effectively if your bloodstream is drip-fed carbs all day – i.e., cereal for breakfast, biscuits with a morning coffee, a sandwich for lunch with a packet of crisps, then a pasta dish with dessert for dinner means you're not using your fat stores as they're intended to be used. Basing a single daily meal on starchy carbohydrates, preferably wholegrain, such as brown oats, brown Basmati rice, quinoa or bulgar wheat achieves the equilibrium we are after. That doesn't mean carbs are banned at other meals, just that they should be in the form of much lighter versions – i.e., sweetcorn, peas, pulses, root veg (carrots, parsnips, new or sweet potatoes, butternut squash) and dairy products.

We are also big fans of protein which should be eaten at every meal because it helps you to feel full quickly and to feel fuller for longer, so you don't feel the need to snack. Remember too that some fat is good for you – it carries fat-soluble vitamins and essential fatty acids that are vital for an ageing body. What we should be avoiding are combinations of fat and sugar or fat and refined flour – the mix you will find in biscuits and pastries, sweets and commercial snack foods. And we haven't jumped on the fruit-shunning bandwagon, preferring instead to alter the effect the natural sugar it contains has on blood glucose by incorporating it into savoury meals.

Fruit is important for providing essential vitamins, minerals, fibre and phytochemicals needed to prevent oxidative damage to cells and inflammation. But by eating it as part of a mixed meal, we get the best of both worlds; a smaller portion combined with other foods leads to a much lower blood sugar rise and it boosts the overall nutrient content of the dish. Fructose (fruit sugar) has the freedom to cause a sugar spike when consumed on its own – and there's inevitably an energy crash that follows. It's that crash that leaves us craving something else and therefore vulnerable to over-eating. This sugar spike is lessened considerably when fruit is combined with healthful grains and leaves. Far better to throw fruit into a salad or tagine than to snack on a single piece between meals.

We are firm believers that we need to move away from the idea that dishes are either sweet or savoury. In reality they can be both. We don't need to have something sweet to follow a savoury dish – that just leads to over-eating. Our philosophy is that if you like fruitcake, don't avoid it, just make it part of a lunch along with some cheese and an apple, spinach and walnut salad. The more foods that are present in one dish, the more slowly they're absorbed for sustained energy. Eating this way will also help realign your taste buds to enjoy the more subtle sweetness of fruit rather than the intense sweetness we have become used to in fizzy drinks and confectionery.

As you've seen, women aged 40 and over generally need to eat fewer calories than is officially recommended, yet we do still require all the vitamins, minerals and other nutrients important for healthy ageing. Our aim is to eat in a way that is nutrient-rich, yet energy-dilute; to get more vitamins for fewer calories. So, we have redefined the food groups to provide a better balance of carbs, protein and healthy fats, while meeting requirements for vitamins and minerals.

Here's what our new recommendations look like:

- ♥ Red meat – 1–2 times a week
- ♥ Other animal non-dairy protein (e.g. chicken and fish) – 1–2 portions a day
- ♥ Plant protein (e.g. soya, nuts, pulses) – 1–2 portions a day
- ♥ Dairy (e.g. cheese, milk, yoghurt) – 2–3 portions a day
- ♥ Colourful fruit and veg (e.g. berries, peppers, tomatoes, melon, mango, pineapple, beetroot) – at every meal

♥ Green and white fruit and veg (e.g. green leafy veg, apples, pears, onions, cucumber, leeks) – at every meal

♥ Starchy veg (e.g. potatoes, sweet potato, root veg, squashes, peas, corn) – at 1–2 meals a day

♥ Whole grains (brown rice, quinoa) – at 1 meal a day

♥ Healthy oils (e.g. avocados, nuts, oils, oily fish) – at 1 meal a day

BOOST YOUR ANTI-AGEING SUPPLIES

The entire ageing process from your first wrinkle to worsening eyesight is affected by oxidation, a process in which damaging free radicals, the body's own exhaust fumes, begin to wear down our DNA. However, promising research has shown that we can slow down ageing in just about every system of our body by eating antioxidant nutrients that offset some of the damage that time and lifestyles inflict on our bodies and minds.

As age starts to take its toll on your skin, the antioxidants in your diet assume more importance than ever. Skin health depends on vitamin C (in fruit and vegetables), betacarotene (in brightly coloured fruit and vegetables) and vitamin E (in avocados and whole grains), as well as essential fatty acids in healthy oils (olive oil and rapeseed oil), nuts and seeds.

Studies by the US government's anti-ageing research department have shown that the amount of antioxidants you maintain in your body is directly proportional to how long you will live [31]. Not all fresh produce packs the same anti-ageing punch. The antioxidant power of food is measured by its ORAC (oxygen radical absorbency capacity) score – the oldest living people consume at least 6000 ORACS a day.

Boosting your ORAC intake

Here is a list of 20 foods that contain 2000 ORAC units. Make sure you dip into the list regularly to keep youth on your side:

- ♥ One-third of a teaspoon of cinnamon
- ♥ Half teaspoon of dried oregano
- ♥ Half teaspoon of turmeric
- ♥ 1 teaspoon mustard
- ♥ Small bowl blueberries
- ♥ Half a pear, grapefruit or plum
- ♥ Small bowl of blackcurrants, raspberries or strawberries
- ♥ Small bowl of cherries
- ♥ An orange or apple
- ♥ 4 pieces of dark chocolate (70% cocoa solids)
- ♥ 7 walnut halves
- ♥ 8 pecan halves
- ♥ Handful of pistachios
- ♥ Lentils
- ♥ ½ tin of kidney beans
- ♥ One-third of an avocado
- ♥ 1 medium bunch broccoli
- ♥ 8 spears of asparagus
- ♥ 150ml (5fl.oz) red wine
- ♥ 200g (7oz) red grapes

CHAPTER FOUR

EXERCISE FOR AN AGELESS BODY

With kids, work, a social life and everything else that eats into your time by midlife, we can reasonably assume that exercise languishes somewhere near the bottom of your pile of priorities. You almost certainly feel you should do more of it, indeed, something at all. Yet trying to squeeze it in can prove impossible some weeks. We know because we've been there. But here's the good news. Compared to the endless hours we both spent working out pre-children, we spend a fraction of that time exercising now. And yet I would wager that, relatively speaking, our fitness levels are on a par with what they were back then.

What's had to change is not just the time we devote to exercise but our perception of what is required to get and stay fit. My background in competitive sport and exercise science coupled with Sarah's own approach to training and the work she has done with elite athletes and professional footballers have given us a colossal bank of experience from which to draw the conclusions that form the basis of our Ageless Body workout plans – namely that it is possible to achieve the body and fitness levels you want in less time than you thought, provided you are prepared to ramp up the effort and be varied with your exercise.

What we've learned is that no single workout approach will achieve all-round benefits as you get older. You need to mix things up, to surprise your body in order to prevent the fitness plateau that results in a physique that looks older than it should. Our plans draw on cutting edge science to target every part of the body and every aspect of physiological fitness. You will be doing elements of the HIIT (high intensity interval training) practised by athletes, along with calisthenics (body weight resistance), weights to offset withering muscles and plain cardio to keep everything ticking over. You will not get bored.

FORGET OFFICIAL GUIDELINES

You'll almost certainly be surprised at how little time you need to devote to exercise for it to take effect. There are huge discrepancies within the fitness industry about how much exercise we really need to be doing on a daily basis just to stay in shape. Depending on where it comes from, the advice on recommended dosage swings from bite-sized chunks being acceptable, to Olympian-style gym sessions being the requirement to improve fitness. Three-minute workouts are a hugely palatable concept for the gym-shy, but others argue we should not be shrinking our activity levels, only increasing them. Take findings presented at the European Congress of Cardiology a few years ago which suggested that cycling fast (or exercising vigorously) for 30–60 minutes a day is the key to avoiding heart problems and living longer [32].

Even the government, a staunch advocate of the 30-minutes-a day approach to activity for many years, has changed its recommendations for adults who should now aim for a minimum

150 minutes a week of moderate exercise – the kind that allows you to enjoy a chat – or 75 minutes of more hardcore stuff, either approach comprising bouts of 10 minutes or more [33]. What's important to distinguish, it seems, is whether you are exercising just to keep things ticking over or whether your aim is to get fitter in a true sense of the word, to hold back the years as much as you can.

Most studies that demonstrate super-mini workouts to be beneficial are focused solely on improving one or more health outcomes. In the case of an occasional '3-minute' sprint every week, for instance, researchers were looking at the activity's influence on insulin sensitivity, the efficiency with which glucose is removed from the bloodstream [34]. It worked, but that's not to say that 3 minutes worth of effort achieves impressive results across the board. Certain physical parameters will improve – your muscle strength and power – but, as with any sort of training, the fitness effects are limited unless you factor in an element of progression.

We've scrutinized the research, consulted the leading exercise scientists and, of course, tried it ourselves to come up with a plan that is both varied and, by necessity, makes you work hard. Our programme won't, however, eat into your lifestyle too much. At the top end, you are looking at 45 minutes a day devoted exclusively to exercise, probably less time than it takes to get the kids ready for school or yourself out the door for a meeting. On some days you will spend as little as 15–20 minutes 'working out'.

There's no denying it will take effort, but we are convinced that the brevity of the sessions and their astounding ability to transform will make it all worthwhile. And let's face it, if you want to achieve anything like the Ageless Body of Helen Mirren, Jennifer Anniston or Halle Berry, it is going to involve some degree of gut-busting.

What we can promise is that, a few weeks in, you'll begin to thrive on the new regimen. What's more, you'll probably wonder why you ever put it off in the first place. It's not just the way it makes you look, but the dramatic effects on your mind and self-confidence that will convince you it is working. Anecdotally, I know dozens of women who claim that the training programme we advocate has helped ease the hormonal turmoil of perimenopausal and menopausal years. It definitely helps me. Mood swings are diminished, sleep is deeper and there are far fewer overly emotional outbursts than I experienced before I stuck to this more varied approach to exercise.

It will also have dramatic effects on your health. Successful ageing is about more than living longer – it's about avoiding debilitating illness past the age of 65, warding off chronic diseases and cognitive decline and, of course, looking and feeling younger. Reams of evidence into the crucial role activity plays in this have emerged, especially in the last five years. Take research from King's College London that clearly showed that active older people resemble much younger people in terms of their health and physiology [35]. A group of men and women aged 55–79 who cycled regularly and fairly seriously but were not competitive athletes, were put through a series of physical and cognitive tests to determine a range of parameters, muscle mass, power, balance, memory skill, bone density and metabolic health among them.

Armed with the results, the researchers compared the statistics with those that are deemed benchmarks of 'normal' ageing. It turned out the active group did not show their age and, in fact, there was little difference between cyclists aged 79 and those aged 55. Those who had continued to exercise in their seventies were as fit as those in their fifties and even the oldest cyclists had the balance ability, reflexes and metabolic health of a youngster. Professor Stephen Harridge, the lead author, said: 'It is not ageing itself which brings about poor function and frailty, but the fact that people have stopped exercising and are no longer active.'

As you will see in Chapter Five, there are endless other anti-ageing benefits to exercise. But suffice to say that the decline in physical health and appearance we once accepted as an inevitability of advancing years is, in fact, largely down to personal choices and decisions. Use it or lose it has never been a more appropriate mantra than it is for the current generation of the middle-aged.

WHY IT'S NEVER TOO LATE TO GET STARTED

All of us can find an excuse not to exercise. There's not enough time, it's too expensive or you just feel too unfit to start. But even if you cancelled your gym membership years ago, haven't pulled on a pair of trainers in months or, indeed, have never 'exercised' in the sense of dedicating time to working out, it's not too late.

I'm what scientists would term an 'ever-exerciser'. There's rarely been a week since the age of 11 when I haven't taken part in sport or a scheduled exercise session. But there are advantages to starting at any age. Believe me, I know women who have taken up running or swimming for the first time in their fifties and sixties and have reaped the benefits. It has rejuvenated their lives and enabled them to rediscover the body that lay beneath the blubber that has been laid down since their more youthful days. There's no reason why you can't aim high just because you took up a fitness programme belatedly.

Scientists have done their bit in offering hope to those who have let their workout habits slip over the past few decades. They have found that taking up exercise in middle age and beyond will greatly improve your long-term health, even if you have previously been a sofa surfer for years. To demonstrate this, a team from the Physical Activity

Research Group at University College, London, trawled through data obtained for the English Longitudinal Study of Ageing, which has tracked the health and fitness habits of tens of thousands of Britons for decades [36]. At the start of the study on a group aged 55–73, they classified the participants as either active (which meant they did an hour or more of activity which was not necessarily 'formal' exercise but could include gardening and walking) or inactive.

After eight years they re-examined their data and re-categorized the subjects according to whether they had stayed active, taken up exercise, remained slothful or had given up activity as they moved beyond middle age. Results, published in the *British Journal of Sports Medicine*, were most encouraging. Those participants who had kept up their activity for the duration of the study had the lowest incidence of chronic disease, memory loss and aches and pains.

But even those who had previously been couch potatoes and had taken up exercise for the first time in their later years reaped considerable rewards in the way of a seven-fold reduction in their risk of becoming ill compared with those who remained in the parked position in front of the TV. In short, the researchers said that older people who exercise at least once a week, no matter when they start, are three to seven times more likely to be classed as 'healthy agers'.

And the beauty of our approach to working out is that it is short, varied and effective. You will not look back.

AGELESS BODY: THE NEW EXERCISE RULES

First things first: Everything you thought you knew about exercising as you get older was probably wrong. Or at least, that much of the previous thinking was flawed when it comes to the best activity for maintaining health, looks and vitality. Taking it all-out easy is not on the cards – you are not yet ready for pushing up daisies. Equally, cardio takes a back seat as exercises previously deemed to be unsuitable for the ageing body – weights, resistance training and intervals – come to the fore.

You will learn much more about the specifics of what you need to do in order to achieve the desired results in Part Two of the book. But, for now, here are the new exercise rules for an Ageless Body:

Increase the intensity: It used to be about how long you spent exercising at the gym, now it's about how little you can get away with. By far the most significant development of working with elite athletes that exercise scientists have bestowed on the masses is the notion that you can spend less time working out if you put in more effort. Believe us, raising the intensity of your activity is not easy. In the beginning you will curse ever having bought this book, but results come quickly and we hope you will be more than satisfied with them.

Make your workouts shorter: If ever there was a woman who epitomized the 'all guns firing' approach to workouts that's been the preserve of female celebrities over the past 10 years, then it was Jennifer Aniston. Here was someone who was known for not just packing her yoga mat when she went on her travels, but her yoga instructor, too. Just reading about her regimen could leave you exhausted. By her own admission she worked out 'almost every day', doing '40 minutes of cardio: spinning, running, the elliptical, or a combination of all three'. Now, in her mid-forties, the former *Friends* star appears to have changed her tune. Of course you should keep active, she said in a recent interview, 'but also take some time off and don't do anything and enjoy your life – I've eased up for sure in the last couple of years'. It has come to something when Aniston says she is cutting back on her exercise, but she isn't the only member of the fitterati to have done so. Gwen Stefani has also announced that she's downsized her regime: 'This past year, I kind of stopped working out,' the 44-year-old admitted. 'I think my body just needed a break. And so I did that and focused more on feeling good as opposed to beating myself up.' And the reason is they know that more is not always better when it comes to working out.

Cut down on distance: A less-is-more philosophy is no more evident than in trends for mass running events. It's one of the reasons why mile races are usurping marathons as the foot-race of choice among those who no longer have the time or inclination to slog out the miles. And attempting shorter distances may be as much of a benefit as doing half marathons, triathlons and the classic 26.2-mile marathon – for your fitness and your appearance. Researchers reporting in the *Journal of the American College of Cardiology* found that, of 55,137 adults, those who ran for less than an hour a week fought off mortality as effectively as runners who were out for three hours a week – with each group out-living non-runners by an average of three years [37]. Really, why slog out more miles than you need to?

Lift weights: Beyond the age of 35, adults lose up to 1lb (0.45kg) of muscle mass a year. Since strength produces the power that is essential for speed, you need to do weights. Encouragingly, a study published in *Medicine & Science in Sports & Exercise* showed that weight training is hugely effective at fighting flab [38]. Forget the old-fashioned belief that it's going to make you bulky. Three groups of women followed an 800-calorie a day diet in addition to either doing no exercise, walking or jogging for up to 40 minutes on a treadmill three times a week, or following an upper and lower bodyweight training session three times a week. All dieted until they lost 25lb (11kg) and both of the exercise groups generally moved more throughout the day, although the weight-trainers more so, thereby burning extra calories and leading to a greater amount of weight loss. An interesting bonus was that weights also led to better walking economy; movement felt easier than before the weight loss and that could transfer to running, too. Proof abounds that weights are well worth the effort.

Become ab-savvy: The mere mention of a bikini or crop top can strike fear into the heart of any women over 25, let alone double that age. Once considered the height of masculinity, gracing only the front covers of *Men's Health*, or the female bodies of those with a Denise Lewis or Jessica Ennis-Hill level of training, the six-pack has become as desirable as cleavage was in the nineties, and has usurped the size zero look of the noughties. Defined abs are everywhere, peeping out beguilingly from crop tops, displayed as a statement of clean living and workout commitment on everyone from athletes to A-listers. We've sought the advice of ab-kings and queens the world over and can inform you that far from being an unrealistic goal, a ripped middle is attainable for the over-forties. What matters is how you go about it and, ironically, endless abdominal exercises (particularly crunches) are out; all-body moves combined with targeted abdominal work are in. It takes time (and effort), but should most certainly not be struck from your agenda prematurely. Prepare to bare, in fact.

Use your body for resistance: Aside from weights (and we're talking dumbbells here, not the hugely expensive kind of equipment you see at the gym), you need no other equipment to achieve a lean and toned physique. In fact, your own body provides the best resistance aid of all and many of the exercises we recommend in Part Two rely solely on moving your own mass. It's a form of training known as calisthenics that, unsurprisingly, has been seized upon by celebrities including Helen Mirren who are living examples of its merits.

Don't get over-bendy: Retaining flexibility is essential at any age, particularly as you get older. But in recent years, a fixation with yoga and related activities that encourage extreme bendiness has taken hold in the belief that the ancient postures alone will help you to achieve the limb length and leanness that portrays yoga. By all means continue with yoga, but please be aware that too much of it can prove detrimental in terms of other aspects of fitness.

I once interviewed the Olympic Cycling gold medallist Victoria Pendleton who told me that she avoided too much flexibility because it had a negative effect on muscle strength and power. And one of the best rejuvenating treatments I've ever experienced was a 'fascial stretching' session with 'stretchpert' Suzanne Waterworth who told me that many of us risk injuring ageing bodies with too much traditional stretching. Where yoga falls down is in its inability to release fascia, the dense, fibrous connective tissue around the body that encompasses all muscles and bones.

In small amounts, fascia is protective, but when it builds up through bad habits, heavy workouts and injury it becomes restrictive, limiting our ability to move freely. Whereas traditional stretching and yoga might increase your suppleness, they won't release fascial tissue. As a result, your body can hold incredible amounts of tension. It's why dancers and yoga addicts are very supple, yet have less stability around their joints leaving them prone to injury. What your body needs is the balance of strength and flexibility outlined in our programme.

Be rested: One of the things you will notice as you get older is that your body needs longer to recover as the years tick by. There are many ways to enhance the recovery process. You can put your feet up and drink sports drinks that aid recovery. You can have a massage or, if you're brave, take an ice bath. Yet the most effective strategy is also the most overlooked: sleep. During deeper sleep, human growth hormone (HGH) produced by the pituitary gland is released into the blood. It is HGH that enables essential recovery processes such as repairing muscles and converting fat to fuel. Consequently, too little sleep means the ageing body produces less HGH and more of the stress hormone cortisol that is an enemy of muscle building and recovery. Recovery experts have become as de rigueur in the world of elite sport as massage therapists, and those I've interviewed are all convinced that we need more recovery as we get older, that perception of effort during a workout is affected when we don't allow ourselves sufficient recovery time – in other words, we think we are working harder when we're sleep-deprived or unrested – as are reaction times, power and other fitness parameters. These are the reasons why our exercise plans schedule in 'active recovery days' as a crucial part of your progress and why we recommend no more than 4–5 days a week of workouts.

Move: A word here about activity, or rather the lack of it. Much of the reason we have slumped unhealthily beyond middle age in recent years is because we spend more time sitting down. Without wishing to scaremonger here, the truth is we have become too lazy for our own good. Collectively, the over-forties are among the most sedentary generation ever and rising inactivity levels affect health as well as appearance. Many of us think we are more active than we are, but tot up the hours you spend on your backside and the chances are they exceed eight a day. We sit down at work, in the car and at home, moving only to shift from one seat to another.

Don't eat to 'fuel' activity: An entire industry has arisen around the concept of needing 'fuel' to complete a workout. Endless energy bars and drinks, gels and packets of pre-workout nuts, seeds and fruit are sold with the claim that they are necessary if you want to avoid crashing and burning mid-session. Unless you are tackling an Olympian-style training regimen, it is simply not the case. For the average person – that's you and me – attempting the kind of workouts outlined in this book, a regular, healthy diet will more than cover the energy output required. Both Sarah and myself are firm believers that you should wipe all notion of 'fueling' and 'refueling' for workout from your mind. They are marketing ploys that will undo the good work you are about to achieve in your Lycra.

Being seated doesn't just burn a bare minimum of calories – even eating an apple or fidgeting uses more energy than parking your bottom on a chair and it is almost inevitable that long-term sitters find their waistlines expanding. Emerging research suggests that there are more sinister happenings when we are inactive for too long. Studies on rats have shown that substances that play a crucial role in metabolising fat and sugar in the body are only produced when muscles are being used, even if that's just standing up. Prolonged sitting has been linked to a sharp reduction in the activity of an important enzyme called lipoprotein lipase which breaks down blood fats and makes them available as a fuel to the muscles. This reduction in enzyme activity leads to raised levels of triglycerides and fats in the blood, increasing the risk of heart disease. Add to that the fact that extended sitting has been shown to cause sharp spikes in blood sugar levels after meals, creating the perfect physiological setting for Type 2 diabetes and it's little wonder we are being urged to get moving.

We are more deskbound than ever before, but do less housework, less shopping, less of everything that involves muscular and cardiovascular effort. Figures from the Royal Automotive Club (RAC) show that total mileage driven is up nearly 20 per cent since 1993. We are laxer around the house, too. A survey of more than 8000 people by Saga attributed the expansion of women's waistlines by 6 inches (15cm) over the past 60 years to them not doing as much housework as their forebears.

Think about it. In the 1950s housewives would burn up to 1000 calories a day simply by doing chores such as washing, mopping and cleaning. The elbow grease required for housework in the 1950s is said to be part of the reason that the average middle-aged woman had a 28-inch (71cm) waist. Today's labour-saving appliances have made life easier, but have cut calorie burning substantially and contributed to the average woman's waistline measurement now being a rather rounder 34 inches (86cm).

Offsetting the risks of inactivity is not easy. Paying a monthly direct debit for gym membership will never count towards our daily activity target unless you actually go to the gym and exercise. Many of us don't bother. One Mintel report suggested that 20 per cent of health club members work out at the fitness emporium – for which they pay a substantial premium – no more than once a month [39].

Even those who are regular gym-goers need to make considerable effort to overcome otherwise lazy lifestyles. When the US National Cancer Institute followed 250,000 adults for eight years to find out how much time they spent exercising, sitting and commuting, they found that those who exercised for 7 hours a week but spent 7 hours a day in front of a TV or computer screen were more likely to die prematurely than those who had less than an hour's daily screen time [40].

The long and short of it is that incidental activity, the kind we used to take in our stride – walking, standing, cleaning, shopping (and, no, not online) – is an essential adjunct to a healthy lifestyle.

We need to move about more in addition to eating healthily and fitting in a daily dollop of a workout. The effects are cumulative and the more incidental activity you can slip into your lifestyle the better the news for your long-term health.

DECADE BY DECADE: WHAT HAPPENS TO YOUR FITNESS?

It's worth looking here at what happens to your body if you don't attempt to stop the free fall with exercise. One of the harsh realities of getting older is that changes to your body take place when you least expect them. Sometimes they are barely noticeable until it becomes apparent that you find things less easy than they used to be, or the aches, pains and niggles after exercise become more persistent and less easy to shake off.

In short, you will begin to find it harder to maintain the basic fitness levels you took for granted in your first few decades of life. The reasons for this are plentiful. Physiological changes in strength and muscle mass, the efficiency of your heart and lungs and the vulnerability of tendons and ligaments can all make exercise feel a bit more like hard work as the years go by. Not everything can be changed. Our goal is to minimize the decline.

What you will find is that recovery from activity also takes longer. Whereas you could once bounce back from a gym session to accomplish another the following day, you will gradually find your body screaming out for longer intervening rest periods as the years go on. In your twenties you likely had higher levels of lean muscle tissue and lower levels of body fat than at any other time in your adult life. This relatively high ratio of calorie burning muscle to fat boosts your metabolism, and made weight maintenance (and loss) relatively easy.

Losing a few extra pounds was no arduous task. I can remember aiming to shed 4–5lbs (2kg) in order to get into an outfit within two weeks and achieving it simply by skipping an occasional meal. Or achieving a flat stomach within two days of cutting out rubbish from my diet. It was no problem and entailed no hardship back then. In my forties, however, I could under-eat for a week and the changes to my body shape would be relatively insignificant.

What science has unearthed and what we have discovered through our own experiments, however, is that although you can't prevent these physiological side effects of ageing, you can slow them down. Do nothing and you can expect the list of adaptations below to occur in what seems an alarmingly accelerated fashion. By changing your exercising habits you can minimize the losses and stem the fitness decline that seemed inevitable.

THIRTIES:

♥ If you've become something of a couch potato – too much 'desk-time', driving or a TV habit – you can begin to lose muscle mass at a rate of 1–2 per cent a year even from the early thirties onwards. This may not sound a lot, but because muscle burns calories, the less lean muscle you have, the less efficiently your body will gobble up the calories you consume. Beware.

♥ On average, your bone mineral density declines at 1 per cent per year from your thirties.

♥ Stress levels often rise during this decade (work, relationships, marriage, kids) and with them comes the release of hormones that increase levels of internal 'visceral' fat laid around the vital organs. You can't see it, but it's there, predisposing your body to a greater risk of heart disease and strokes and making a fitness regimen imperative.

♥ Gaining weight in your thirties can hamper fertility if you are trying to get pregnant.

FORTIES:

♥ It suddenly requires a lot more diligence to maintain body tone. This is because muscle loss occurs at its fastest rate in the mid-forties and is down by 4–7lbs (2–3kg) compared with a decade ago.

♥ Weight creeps on, often imperceptibly at first. You need, on average, 145 fewer calories per day at 45 than you did at 25.

♥ In addition, your metabolism also begins to slow by 2 per cent per decade from now on, which is why the forties are the decade in which we are most likely to notice middle age spread.

♥ From the age of 40 onwards, maximal aerobic capacity, the efficiency with which your body can use oxygen, begins to drop steadily, declining by as much as 10 per cent per decade.

♥ Your kidneys conserve water less effectively, meaning you are more prone to dehydrating in an endurance challenge like the marathon.

♥ Wear and tear on the joints is more pronounced, and recovery also takes longer. Tired, over-used muscles simply don't repair themselves as quickly as they did when they were springy and youthful.

FIFTIES:

♥ You'll start to notice aches and niggles. It might be occasional at first – when you get up in the morning, when you stand up after being sat at a desk for hours. Muscles and ligaments are no longer as pliable as they used to be and require upkeep.

♥ Joints also become stiffer with age. Dr Ceri Diss, an exercise scientist at the University of Roehampton, has found that ankle stiffness is a key factor in slowing down runners and walkers in their fifties [41]. The ankle is the joint that changes the most with age; stiffness means it doesn't absorb the shock of a running stride very effectively and it reduces the ability to exert power in a running or walking stride.

♥ With oestrogen levels beginning to drop, many women find they begin to gain around 1lb (0.5kg) a year from now until they reach the menopause at the average age of 52.

♥ Where did those bulges appear from? Female fat distribution changes most dramatically between the ages of 40 and 55, with many women finding they become a classic 'apple' shape.

♥ You need 200 fewer calories a day than you did in your twenties.

DID YOU KNOW?

A study of post-menopausal women in the European Journal of Applied Physiology showed that after swimming twice a week for 24 weeks, they were able to complete an average 28 more abdominal crunches than when they started. They also experienced a 15 per cent reduction in body fat and an 8 per cent drop in blood pressure [42].

SIXTIES:

♥ Try to run 5km with someone half your age and, unless you have been training like a pro, you'll struggle even if they are seemingly less fit. Your maximal oxygen uptake (which influences your aerobic fitness) is down by as much as one third, on average, compared with people of 25. Good news is that your endurance capacity does not drop as dramatically – provided you keep up aerobic activity.

♥ From this age onwards, expect to lose up to 0.4 inches (1cm) a year in height due to muscle and other tissue loss unless you address the issue with a targeted programme.

♥ Flexibility and elasticity of muscles, ligaments and joints declines, even further affecting power and speed.

♥ The shift to more of an 'apple shape' as weight moves to the midriff signals that someone also possesses more visceral fat (positioned around the organs), the type that promotes heart disease and inhibits glucose tolerance, a precursor for diabetes.

SEVENTIES:

♥ 'But I used to be 5 feet 7 inches....' Height loss accelerates to as much as 1.2 inches (3cm) a year in some people and can lead to kyphosis (the medical term for a hunched back) which can affect ease of breathing and result in neck pain.

♥ By this decade, the average person has lost 25 per cent of their muscle mass compared with when they were in their thirties.

♥ One woman in three suffers the bone thinning disease osteoporosis by this age.

DID YOU KNOW?

Texas University researchers found that resistance training for six months improved the sleep quality as well as fitness levels of 70-year-olds by an average 38% [43].

EIGHTIES:

♥ Your muscles, liver, kidney and other organs lose some of their cells – a process called atrophy.

♥ Water content is also lost from all of the body's structures, including the cartilage that protects joints.

♥ Tissues become weaker and less compliant.

♥ Your metabolism slows and you require a lower calorie intake.

DID YOU KNOW?

A study at the University of South Florida divided volunteers with an average age of 84 into three groups to test the effects of activity. While one group exercised by walking, the second did weight training and the third group did no exercise. After four months both of the exercise groups had lower blood pressure, improved body strength, better flexibility and higher scores in tests of balance and coordination compared with their sedentary counterparts [44].

WHAT ABOUT GYM FACE?

Reach a certain age and there comes a tipping point with weight loss that begins to make you wonder if it's all worthwhile. 'I'd love to run a marathon/hike the Pyrenees/compete in an Ironman, but exercise just adds years to my face' is among the most common cry among female friends of mine who have begun shunning the gym in a bid to preserve their visage.

And they have a point. Let's be honest, we all know someone who has gym face. Not only does she avoid carbs and dairy, but she is your fitness queen, barely spotted sans-Lycra and skipping like a greyhound around local fun runs, but adding a decade or so to her appearance in the process. She has achieved enviable leanness, but the price to pay is drawn features, sunken cheeks and hollow eyes.

Endurance activities beloved of this age group are the main culprit, partly because they cause dramatic weight loss but also inflict the kind of prolonged wear and tear that exacerbates a drop in skin's youthful plumpness. Think about it – spend hours in the gym or pounding the pavements in your running shoes and of course you will see fat melt away from your middle-age spread, but also from the place you least want to lose plumpness in your late thirties and onwards: your face.

Add the hormonal desert of the menopause (and the drop in oestrogen which causes facial muscles to slacken) and it's hardly surprising that hordes of women abandon the excessive back-to-back cardio and weights workouts that led to the sinewy and gaunt look that Madonna flaunted a decade ago.

Cosmetic surgeons in the UK report a 20 per cent rise in recent years of the middle aged paying for dermal fillers, designed to fill any deep crevices in the skin and increase lost volume, alongside Botox, to iron out the wrinkles that accompany facial fat loss. It's a drastic attempt to claw back youthful looks, but there's an easier and healthier way to retain the bloom of youth without storing fat where you don't want it. For scientists have proven that opting instead for a more face-friendly fitness regimen can pay dividends. And it won't surprise you to learn that it's exactly what we recommend in the Ageless Body plans.

Our mix of shorter bursts of higher intensity exercise along with resistance exercise and some aerobic activity is the perfect recipe for anti-ageing. Indeed, the American Council on Exercise, a not-for-profit organization that commissions studies and collates evidence on the benefits and otherwise of activity, states: 'There is a tremendous amount of evidence to suggest that high intensity strength training and cardiorespiratory exercise can be the stimulus to produce numerous anti-ageing benefits' [50]. Strength training, using either weights or your own body with exercises such as squats and lunges, is also crucial as it promotes muscle protein synthesis for building new muscle cells and keeping skin all over the body taut and toned. And while occasional long runs or cycles are perfectly fine, we generally go with the science that suggests anything over 75 per cent of maximum effort for longer than 45 minutes on a regular basis is a recipe for gym face at 45-plus.

Let's just consider the benefits that the right kind of exercise can have on your appearance. Scientists at McMaster University in Ontario tested this in a trial that was not your routine scientific experiment [46]. They recruited 29 volunteers aged 20–84, half of whom took part in about three fitness sessions a week while the others did only about an hour of activity in total. Each volunteer was asked to bare a buttock so that skin least likely to be damaged by sun exposure could be analysed. Samples were then taken and after carrying out biopsies, the scientists divided them according to age and exercise habits, then examined the stratum corneum (the skin's protective outermost layer) and the dermis layer underneath.

Typically, most people begin to experience a thickening of the stratum corneum, which is laden with dead skin cells, after 40. It also begins to sag, droop and wrinkle. With diminishing elasticity, the dermis gets thinner and turns somewhat translucent. Yet the scientists found that the regular exercisers had significantly thinner and healthier stratum corneum and thicker dermis layers after the age of 40. Some in their forties had skin biopsies expected in those half their age and the effects persisted even past age 65. The findings support research by scientists at the Saarland University Clinic in Germany who, while looking at cell lifespans of experienced middle-aged runners (who didn't cover excessive distances) versus sedentary peers, noted how much younger the joggers looked [47]. In the McMaster trial it seemed that skin composition was partly boosted by raised levels in the bloodstream of protein substances called myokines. Levels of one, called IL-15, soared by almost 50 per cent in the skin samples tested after the exercise programme.

So, what we know is that exercise can – indeed will – lead to a more youthful appearance provided it's the right sort of activity. Through our own experimentation, both Sarah and I have found the happy medium: exercise that gets you fit, healthy and toned without leaving you looking as if you have fast-forwarded your face through the decades.

In the next chapter we look at some of the more unexpected highlights of our diet and exercise regimen and how, ultimately, it might add years to your life.

CHAPTER FIVE

THE AGELESS BODY AND LONGEVITY

One of the things that strikes with force when you reach 40 and beyond is a sense of mortality. I have friends for whom this very notion becomes a source of overwhelming doom, a fear so pronounced that it seems to affect their enjoyment of life in every respect. There is nothing we can do to prevent the inevitable; we all, sooner or later, shuffle off the mortal coil. But wallowing in that realization won't help us. How we live has been proven to postpone the appearance of the Grim Reaper, to enhance longevity. And diet along with exercise play the most significant of roles in helping this to happen.

For, while the Ageless Body plan can make you look and feel better, there's another welcome knock-on effect: you could live longer as a result of following it. A diet replete in vegetables, healthy grains and nuts and one that allows for periods of fasting has been proven to lengthen the lifespan of both animals and humans in trials. Coupled with the right kind of exercise, the outcome can be so significant that even my age-weary friends can't help but feel uplifted by the prospect of gaining a good few extra years on this planet.

Respected experts are spreading the word. Professor Sir Muir Gray, the former chief of knowledge for the National Health Service (NHS) has said that instead of spending more time in an armchair, even those in their sixties, seventies and eighties should be working out in order to prolong their lives. Speaking at the Oxford Literary Festival in 2015, Sir Muir said 'we should have a bonfire of slippers' to ensure the elderly remain fit and healthy, advocating dumbbells as an ideal gift for grandparents and elderly relatives, and suggesting 'the number one present for people aged 70 should be resistance bands. They should be standard' [48].

We are a generation that should be looking with cheeriness, not dread, towards many more birthdays than our grandparents enjoyed, simply by overhauling the way we live on a daily basis. Here are some of the highlights you can expect to happen when you do:

Your heart: In addition to a healthy diet with none of the nasties that clog up your arteries, exercise, in any form, will boost the health of your heart. What's intriguing scientists lately is how little activity you need to do in order to achieve a younger-acting ticker. Short duration, high intensity exercise combined with the good old heart health favourite, aerobic activity, seems to be the most clear-cut route to staving off heart disease in later life.

Dr John Babraj, from the University of Abertay's School of Social and Health Sciences, showed that just two 60-second workouts a week can reduce heart disease risk from middle age onwards. Each session consisted of 6-second all-out sprints on an exercise bike with the number of sprints progressively increased over the course of the trial, from six to ten. On average, his subjects lost 2lbs (1kg) of fat in a two-month trial even though they didn't change their diet or activity habits in other ways. They also had significantly better cardiovascular function, an important marker of heart disease, after eight weeks [49].

In short, your forties are not a time for slowing down. Whatever you do, do it harder, is our motto. Take a Danish study in the British Medical Journal that looked at more than 10,000 adults. It found a daily power-walk or jog was found to curb the risk of heart disease by as much as 50 per cent, whereas a slow amble made little overall difference. Fast walking was found to halve the risk of metabolic syndrome – a combination of factors including a bulging midriff, high blood pressure and abnormal blood-fat levels, all of which are risks for heart disease – whereas jogging reduced the risk by 40 per cent [50]. It's a no brainer that the kind of workouts we advocate in our plan are going to maintain your heart health for longer.

Your joints: Exercise gets a pretty bad rap when it comes to the ageing of your joints. It's widely assumed that 'pounding' activities are about as good for your knees as taking a hammer to the joint and hitting it. Yet it's not as straightforward as that. Exercise in itself is often not the root cause of joint pain. Poor technique, a lack of variety in your sport and previous injuries can predispose you to osteoarthritis in later life, as can being overweight (the major cause). Indeed, physical activity is crucial for keeping your joints mobile and even deterring joint conditions such as arthritis, a scourge of the middle aged. Professor Sir Muir Gray says prescribing exercise for conditions like arthritis could be 'far better than most medications people are on'.

What works for joint protection is surprising. While non-weight bearing activities such as swimming and cycling are kind to the joints, even some high impact sports can have huge benefits. Running, for example, is now seen as less risky than sports like football and tennis, even offering protection to vulnerable joints. Indeed, a team from Stanford University's division of immunology and rheumatology found that adults who run consistently can expect to have 25 per cent less osteoarthritis and musculoskeletal pain than non-runners when they get older [51]. Protection from running was in part linked to greater muscle strength and healthier bones and connective tissues, but experts suspect it is also the fact that running is in one direction, with no twisting and turning, that could make it more joint-friendly.

Work at Loughborough University is looking at the effects of different types of strength training on recovery from sports injuries. So far, the sports scientist Dr Jonathan Folland has shown that fast, explosive weight training produces more benefits than conventional strength exercise after four weeks. With rehabilitation, says Folland, the aim is to increase stiffness of muscles and tendons, which not only improves function but reduces the risk of further injury, as they are more robust, less easily overstretched and damaged.

A nutrient-rich diet that doesn't pile on the pounds is also essential. Dr James Bilzon, an exercise physiologist at the University of Bath who is working with the Rugby Football Union Injured Players' Foundation, says low-grade joint inflammation can be well managed through diet. His trials aim to show the effects of vitamin D and omega-3 acid supplementation to see whether it can help before and after injury.

Professor Mark Batt, a consultant in sport and exercise medicine at Nottingham University Hospitals and the director of the Arthritis Research UK Centre for Sport, Exercise and Osteoarthritis which combines the expertise of specialists in sports medicine and osteoarthritis at many of the top UK universities, says that whatever you do, eat well and try to keep moving.

Exercise, he says, is always a positive thing for joints; being active far outweighs the risks associated with the kind of injury that might eventually progress into osteoarthritis. 'The aim of our research centre is to find out ways to help all active people prevent or slow down degeneration of their joints,' Professor Batt says. 'We want to keep people active for as long as we can.'

Libido: Friskiness is too often considered age dependent. As female hormones ebb and flow, so the libido must follow suit. Says who, we'd like to know? Neither of us has noticed a downturn in our respective bedroom antics and, thankfully, the received wisdom that age dampens desire is challenged by studies that show sexual desire can be boosted, whatever your age.

A sure-fire way to get your flagging mojo back is through exercise. Multiple studies have also shown that after just 20 minutes of exercise, blood flow to the genitals increases, resulting in more lubrication, better arousal and, hoorah, better orgasms. It's good news. One trial conducted at the University of Texas at Austin went as far as proving that female sex drive may actually increase as a woman's sex hormones and fertility decrease [52]. Two more studies from Harvard University measured the increase in libido after regular exercise in both college students and people aged 40–60. Without exception, the more physically vigorous subjects reported a higher incidence of sexual activity [53]. Elsewhere, researchers at the University of Arkansas reported that 60 per cent of women who exercised two to three times per week rated their sex appeal as 'above average' [54].

Among women who have been prescribed antidepressants, the effects are particularly pronounced. Moderate exercise activates the sympathetic nervous system, which plays a role in blood flow to the genital region. Antidepressants have been shown to depress this system, but researchers at Indiana University found that depressed women who did 30 minutes of exercise immediately before sex experienced a significant boost in libido and overall improvements in sexual functioning [55]. Working out will also keep your weight down, another compounding factor for your libido. The more your percentage of body fat rises as you get older, the less libido-boosting 'free-floating' testosterone you have. For the very overweight and obese, a 10 per cent drop in fat can boost your sex drive, found researchers at Duke University [56].

Blood sugar: What you eat has a direct impact on your blood sugar status and, consequently, on your long-term risk of diabetes. Consume high amounts of sugary foods or refined carbohydrates on a daily basis and your blood sugar levels can rise rapidly. Not only can this cause feelings of stress and anxiety, but it can disrupt your body's ability to control blood glucose levels. As the pancreas is put under pressure to manufacture huge amounts of insulin needed to control blood sugar, cells become resistant to its effects, eventually giving rise to the killer condition.

Not all foods have this effect. Blood sugar levels adapt positively to the low GI foods, the kind that release their energy slowly, which is why you will be eating plenty of them on our plan. Cutting out snacks, as we recommend, also means that there are no sharp rises in your blood glucose level followed by the big dip which leaves you feeling tired and drained. Exercise also helps, in particular the high intensity kind. In Dr Babraj's trials on the effects of just two short workouts a week on a group of middle-aged people, measures of blood sugar control showed improvements almost matching those of younger people doing more of the same exercise [57].

Brain power: It starts with forgetting where the keys are, but can end up with you forgetting where you live. Memory loss and its associated conditions are among the most feared of all side effects of ageing. So any means of halting (or better still, preventing) cognitive decline are welcomed as we enter the second half of life. What's clear from the research that has been conducted in this area (and there's a lot of it) is that what is good for the heart, also seems to be beneficial for the brain. And remaining physically active is perhaps the most important step you can take in protecting your grey matter from ageing.

Many studies have documented benefits to the brain from regular exercise. Among the most compelling results are those obtained from the Nurses Health Study at Harvard University in which 18,766 women aged 70 to 81 were questioned about their activity levels. Those who did the most exercise were one-fifth less likely to suffer cognitive impairment than the inactive [58].

Brain-friendly foods include antioxidant-rich vegetables and fish along with plenty of vitamin D, whereas those foods more likely to dull your memory are high in fats (particularly the chemically altered trans fats) – in one study at the University of California, San Diego School of Medicine, each gram of trans fats eaten per day was associated with 12 to 21 fewer words recalled, out of an average score of 86 [59] – and the Devil's candy, aka sugar.

Using laboratory rats trained to find their way out of a maze, researchers at the University of California, Los Angeles, found that when some animals were fed a fructose solution and others plain water for six weeks, the sugar eaters forgot the escape route [60]. According to the scientists at the UCLA Brain Research Institute, the memory loss in the sugar-consuming rats was triggered by an onset of insulin resistance caused by their prolonged high intake of the sugary drink. In time, it damaged their synapses – the connections between brain cells that enable learning.

So what does maintain memory? A five-year study involving almost 30,000 people from 40 countries, published in the journal *Neurology*, found that those who consumed the most fruit and vegetables, nuts and soy proteins, whole grains and a higher ratio of fish to meat and eggs in their diet were 24 per cent less likely to have experienced cognitive decline than those who ate less healthy diets that included fast and processed foods [61].

Among the 5687 healthier eaters, around 14 per cent had cognitive decline compared with about 18 per cent of the 5459 people with the least healthy diets. The results were the same when researchers accounted for other factors like physical activity, high blood pressure and history of cancer. All of which goes a long way to support the diet we have prescribed as healthy for body as well as for mind.

So much for the science and theory. In Part Two we look at how you can implement the changes in your own life so that an Ageless Body becomes reality. We discuss what to eat and when, how much to exercise and what type of activity to do. It's time to develop your action plan.

PART TWO

As we've seen, there are plenty of scientifically sound reasons to embark on our programme of exercise and eating plan with 4-hour fasting as its core principle. Follow it and you are likely to lower your blood pressure, cholesterol levels and, of course, your percentage body fat. Above all you will begin to regain the body shape and health of someone much younger. So, with the theory out of the way, it's time to get down to the nitty-gritty of the Ageless Body plan and how to introduce it into your own life. It's your turn to do the work.

CHAPTER SIX

HOW TO USE THIS BOOK

WHEN TO GET STARTED

What's wrong with right now? What we've discovered through both our own experiences and interviews with hundreds of women is that the older you get, the more reasons there are not to make positive switches to your lifestyle. Too time crunched, too stressed and too flaming exhausted are the most common reasons we come across. Yet we urge you to take the plunge, not least because you are likely to find most of these draining negativities will be overturned.

A huge draw of the Ageless Body plan is that it is designed to be followed for the rest of your life. It is by no means a short-term fix and won't cause the unwelcome side effects so often associated with other diet and exercise regimens. We have all experienced the gnawing hunger, the mood lows and the overwhelming fatigue that can accompany a fast track approach to weight loss. But this book is about more than that. Sure, you will shed pounds, likely drop a dress size or more, but the most staggering difference will be to your body confidence and your vitality levels.

As with any new diet and activity programme, there are some precautions you should take before you start, particularly if you haven't exercised in a while. Have a once-over health check from your GP to make sure everything is in order (I now make an annual appointment to check blood cholesterol levels, blood pressure and everything else). Of course, if you have an underlying medical issue you should not attempt any new plan unless it's been approved by your nurse or specialist.

It's also worth remembering that the advice is tailored to those of us who are over 35 years of age. While the meals can be consumed by the whole family, there are aspects of the plan that we certainly don't advocate for children. While they are growing (which continues until they are 19 or 20 in some cases), children need a regular supply of top-notch nutrients. Contrary to the studies that have been conducted on adults, regular meals including breakfast are important for youngsters. Likewise, prescribed exercise is not recommended for the under-11s and children should be encouraged to engage in as much 'incidental' activity as they can through play and games. There is no reason why you can't join in, of course.

In summary, there really is no time like the present to get going. Here's to your very own Ageless Body.

WHEN TO EAT

Now we are down to the business end of your preparation. How easy it is to adjust to the eating patterns we recommend depends on what your current diet looks like. It's by no means essential, but you might find it helpful to take a week to analyse how and why you eat at the moment. Jot down in a journal when you consume food and drink, logging everything from your first coffee of the day to the muffin or biscuit you have mid-morning and the nuts you nibble at your desk.

If you can, write down why you ate. Were you hungry or bored? Did you feel you needed an energy boost? Was that bowl of breakfast cereal eaten out of habit or because you really couldn't face the day without something in your stomach? Be brutally honest, as it will give you much more of an idea as to how best to schedule your Ageless Body plan. Once you've had a long hard look at your eating habits you can begin to plan your Ageless Body eating schedule.

Meals can be eaten when you like as long as you keep to the 4 hour or more gap in between. On average this will mean that you are aiming for two to three meals a day. But if you are a very early riser who also goes to bed late, then your extended day means you can feasibly fit in an extra meal with the allotted 4-hour break. So, if your first meal is at 7.30 a.m., you could have a bowl of soup at around midday, another bowl at 4 p.m. and then supper at 8 p.m. We are certainly not expecting you to starve.

The 4-hour rule may seem tough at first, especially if you are a confirmed snacker, so focus on ways to change your habit of opening the fridge every time you go into the kitchen. Start by deciding whether or not you need to eat breakfast. Cutting out that first meal of the day isn't as drastic as it sounds. It might be that you eat one of our breakfast suggestions later in the morning, in which case you may not feel like lunch, or you may prefer to skip breakfast completely and go through until lunch, but you will need to make lunch slightly more substantial.

HOW TO EAT

Our four-week diet plan is designed to maximize satisfaction and minimize hassle. It works in tandem with the four-week exercise plans and can be repeated or adapted as you progress through the various stages of the workout regimens. Our aim is that, within a month or so of switching to our proposed way of eating, you will become so hooked on the effects that you'll be more than adept at sticking to the philosophy.

All of our daily menus are flexible and you can mix and match some of our suggestions according to what else you eat. By all means pick and mix your meals depending on what you have time for or what you have in the fridge. But try to remember the 'one heavy carb meal a day' rule. This means if you are having the berry porridge for breakfast, avoid the oatcakes for lunch; instead, choose something much lighter in carbs.

Take Monday in week one, for example. You might choose to have the smoothie at 11 a.m. with a couple of the oatcakes and peanut butter. By 3 p.m. have a few more of the allotted oatcakes with the cottage cheese, pear and walnuts. Or if you don't want to eat until lunchtime, have the oatcakes and cottage cheese, pear and walnuts and add a yoghurt with some berries or sliced banana. If you miss breakfast on Tuesday, add a dollop of yoghurt to your soup and serve with a toasted wholemeal pitta.

We have opted for larger brunch-style meals at weekends, assuming that you may have more time and be willing to try something a bit more adventurous. But this doesn't hold for everyone and you can substitute a weekend meal for a weekday if you prefer. A larger brunch followed by no lunch (Peta's preferred approach) allows you to indulge in a more hearty evening meal, so weekend suppers tend to be more filling and worth the effort. And don't forget to make use of the comprehensive shopping lists we have included as they should make it much easier for you to avoid mindless eating and to help you minimize waste.

WHAT TO EAT

One thing you don't have to worry about is getting sufficient nutrients – this plan is rammed with what you need to stay healthy as you get older. Nutrient demands on your body change with advancing years and we've ensured that you get enough of everything required to look and feel younger than you really are. Neither of us are huge fans of supplements, taking them only when we feel we have let things slip a little (we are all human). Instead we prefer to obtain micronutrients from as natural a source as possible: food. Here's an idea of what you'll be consuming by the week:

Iron-rich foods: Your menstrual cycle is likely to become erratic as you get older. Many women approaching the menopause experience heavier periods than they have during other times of their lives, the upshot of which is you could very easily become anaemic. The signs of iron deficiency anaemia – lethargy, listlessness, inability to concentrate – are frequently ignored because we think it's just how life is making you feel. But boosting your natural iron levels is very important and can be easily achieved through diet.

Red meat is the best source of the most easily absorbed form of iron called 'haem-iron', but eggs, beans, pulses and whole grains are also rich in iron, which is why they feature prominently in our plan. We've also included plenty of vitamin C-rich foods like peppers, kiwi fruit and tomatoes as they help to increase your absorption of the iron from other foods.

Antioxidants: As age starts to take a toll on your skin, the antioxidant vitamins A, C and E in your diet have taken on more importance than ever. Skin health depends on vitamin C (found in fruit and vegetables), betacarotene (in brightly coloured fruit and vegetables) and vitamin E (in avocados and whole grains), as well as essential fatty acids in healthy oils (olive oil and rapeseed oil), nuts and seeds. All are in plentiful supply in our recipes.

Phytoestrogens: Studies have shown that you can help balance your hormone levels by eating foods rich in plant oestrogens such as soya, lentils and chickpeas and linseeds. In Asia, where the average woman's daily intake of isoflavones is 20–80mg a day (in the form of tofu, miso and soy sauce or lentils), perimenopausal symptoms are only reported by 14 per cent. But in the West, where our isoflavone intake is a paltry 1–3mg per day, the same symptoms affect 80–85 per cent of women. It makes sense to boost your intake of phytoestrogens in a natural way – through food rather than relying on supplements.

Oats: By adding soluble fibre to your diet in the form of oats and pulses, you can help to lower your cholesterol levels. Soluble fibre works by binding bile acids in the gut so they cannot then be reabsorbed into the body. More cholesterol is needed to make the new bile acids, so leaving less swimming around in the blood. Both of us are avid fans of porridge, oatcakes and pulses so you will find plenty of recommendations for these age-defying ingredients.

Essential fats: Thankfully, the idea that all fat is unhealthy has been rebuffed by recent science. We now know for definite that not all fats are bad and that some have a hugely positive influence on our bodies and minds. These healthy fats found in oils, nuts, seeds and avocados effectively help to 'oil' the ageing body by lubricating the joints. They also improve your complexion, help to balance hormones, insulate nerve cells and keep arteries supple. In addition they can boost the metabolism and help with weight loss. High fat foods like avocados should be your diet staples.

Fish oils: There's plenty of science showing that the long-chain omega-3 fats in fish oils also help to reduce all sorts of harmful inflammatory processes that accelerate ageing. So many common ageing symptoms such as dry hair, dry skin, cracked nails, fatigue, depression, lack of motivation and even aching joints stem from a deficiency of essential fatty acids.

Vitamin D: The body's ability to synthesize vitamin D from sunlight is reduced with age and if you find yourself spending less time outdoors than you used to, you could end up with less vitamin D than you need. Vitamin D plays an important role in helping the absorption of calcium, but it is also implicated in your immunity, so boosting vitamin D could reduce your cancer risk. Oily fish, cheese, eggs and mushrooms are all good sources.

Get your greens: Leafy green vegetables such as kale, broccoli, Brussels sprouts, pak choi, spinach, chard, okra and asparagus are a powerhouse of good stuff for women as they get older. They contain folate needed for healthy blood and potassium to help regulate blood pressure, and are rich in soluble fibre, which helps boost good gut bacteria and reduce systemic inflammation, a condition that increases your risk of immune disorders, aches and pains and even heart disease. Boosting your intake of these vegetables also helps your body make vitamin K and helps maintain bone density by increasing your body's production of oestocalcin, a protein that strengthens bones.

Be fruity: We are firmly against the current trend for avoiding fruit because of its natural sugar content. Instead we advocate adding it to savoury meals which will lower its glycaemic index (or GI), satisfy a sweet tooth and provide heaps of other benefits. Berries are low in sugar and packed full of antioxidants, particularly vitamin C, which is needed for the production of collagen, an important protein for maintaining good skin. They contain high levels of anthocyanins, a type of flavonoid that is believed to help dilate arteries, reduce the build-up of plaque in arteries and offer other cardiovascular benefits. All fresh fruits are rich in potassium which also helps regulate blood pressure and maintain healthy fluid balance.

WHEN TO EXERCISE

There are no hard and fast rules as to the best time of day to exercise. It comes down to when you feel best and, of course, when you can fit it into your day. The beauty of the Ageless Body workout plans is that they don't require huge chunks of time and slip easily into your routine. What's more, recovery of muscles takes longer as we get older, so more rest is needed between sessions. That is why we have limited the number of workouts to four a week with the option of adding a further session if you really feel you need it as you get further into the plan.

We have found from personal experience (and from interviewing dozens of women about their exercise habits) that it helps to pre-schedule in your workout and not rely on some opportune moment arising – more often than not it simply won't happen. There's some evidence that we are more suited to exercise at certain times of the day than at others. A study at Glasgow University reported that a morning workout leads to a bigger reduction in artery-clogging blood fats [62]. Evidence also showed that getting up with the lark might make a workout feel more difficult, but it is a more effective route to mood-boosting throughout the day.

According to the Glasgow researchers, who published their findings in the journal *Appetite*, women completing an 8.15 a.m. aerobics class achieved a 50 per cent increase in positive thoughts compared with those who postponed their workout until 7.15 p.m.

But evenings suit some people better. Researchers at Liverpool John Moores University found this to be the case among a group of people they asked to exercise at different times of day [63]. Most felt the 5 a.m. session to be far more of a slog than the 5 p.m. session. Elite swimmers, who train notoriously early in the day, have been shown to have a 10–15 per cent drop in performance first thing. Body temperature rises throughout the day, meaning that your muscles are more primed for activity between 12 and 7 p.m. even if your mind is saying no. Beware though that this reverses from early evening onwards and that an intense workout directly before bed has been found to hamper sleep patterns in some people.

With almost as much research supporting an early workout as a late one, ultimately it comes back to personal preference. I've found that my approach has changed over the years. In my twenties and thirties (pre-children and pre-mortgage), I was more than happy to get up before everyone else for my exercise. Now I can barely drag myself out of bed if I try, preferring to work out either after the school run in the morning or at around 2–3 p.m. when my joints feel more agile and my conscience is eased by the fact that at least I have managed to accrue some work to pay the bills. And any time is better than none at all.

HOW TO EXERCISE

We've made the exercise plans as self-explanatory as possible. Before each we advocate a brief warm-up. This needn't be anything extravagant, but it's not a great idea to go straight from sitting on the sofa into a high intensity session (or any form of exercise for that matter). A few minutes of easing the body gently into workout mode does the trick and I prefer a gentle jog, walking on the spot or some skipping.

If you feel better for a stretch, then by all means do some flexibility exercises before you start. Evidence suggests that static stretching (the kind in which you hold a position for several seconds) has less of a positive effect on performance than once thought and may even impact negatively on strength work that follows. That may be the case, but I personally feel my body is better prepared after I've flexed the hamstrings that have become tightened through endless sitting at my desk.

If you mix your workouts, try to stick to performing the prescribed workouts on non-consecutive days as much as possible. This is not a strict rule, but helps the body recover which, in turn, means you are less likely to quit midway through the week. On days when no specific workout is allocated, it is not a signal for you to be bone-idle. As we have seen, too much sitting is a sure route to middle age bumps and bulges, the very thing we are trying to avoid. Keep as active as possible, walking when you could drive, cycling when you could take the bus, playing in the park with the kids when you could sit on the bench and watch. Make activity part of your lifestyle and the Ageless Body will be that much easier to achieve and maintain.

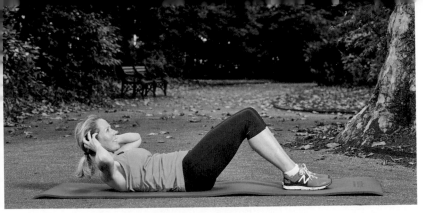

Crunch: these form an important part of any abs-toning routine

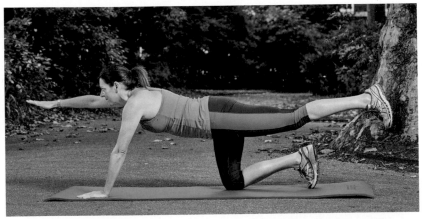

Superman: performing these in a controlled manner works the abs, bottom and lower back

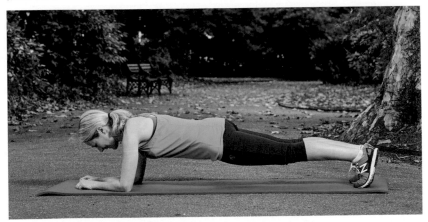

Plank: make sure sure your body is in as straight a line as possible

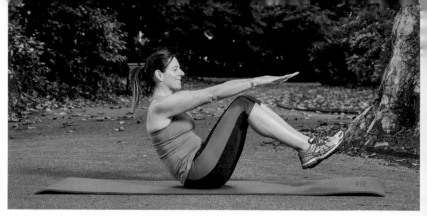

V-sit: these are tough but really get results

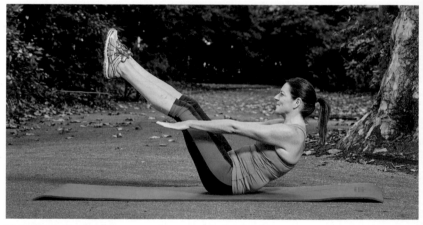

V-sit alternative: straighten your legs to work even harder

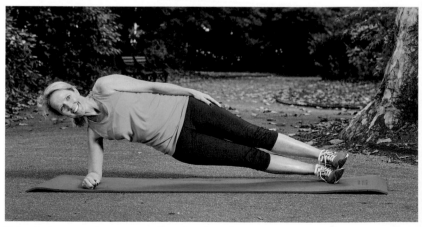

Side plank: concentrate on not dropping those hips

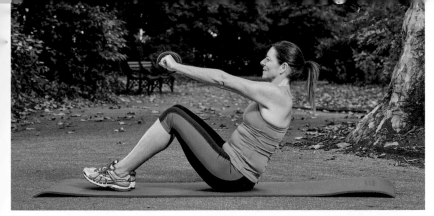

Russian twist start position

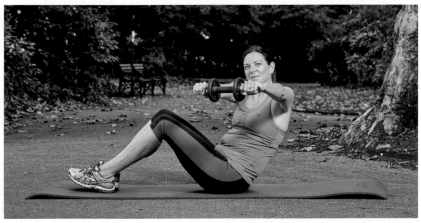

Russian twist: keep your head up and eyes forward to help with balance

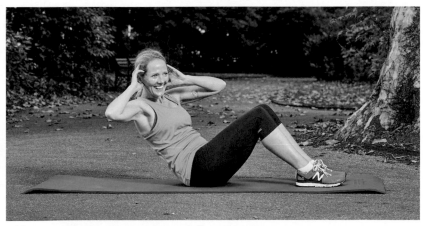

Oblique crunch: this one focuses on working the waist

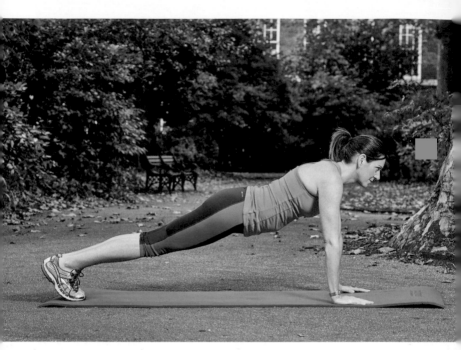

Above: Press-up start position; *below:* Press-up

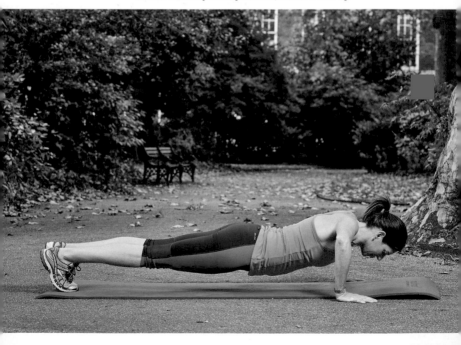

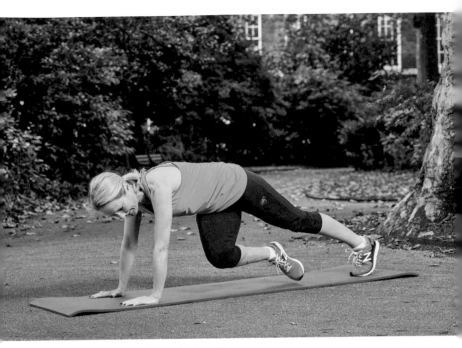

Above and below: Knee crossovers

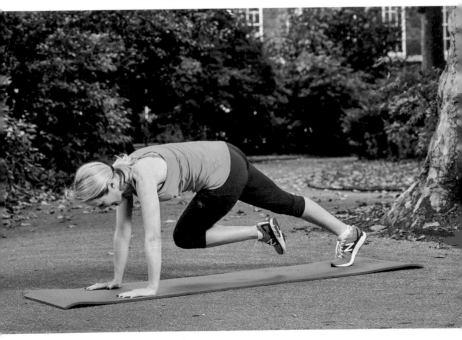

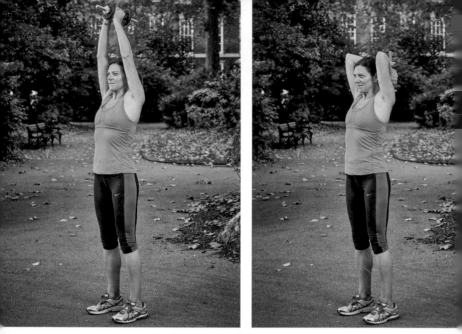

Left and right: Triceps extension

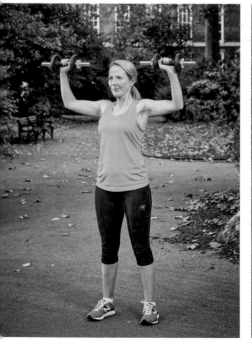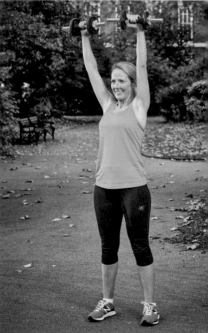

Left and right: Shoulder press

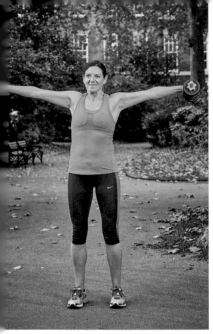

Lateral raise

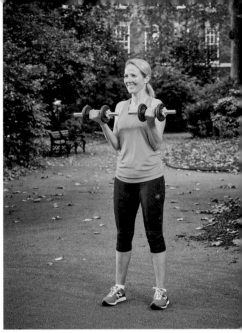

Bicep curl

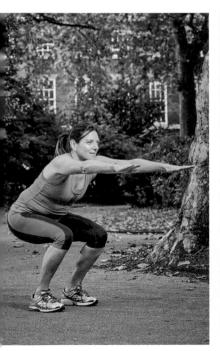

Squat

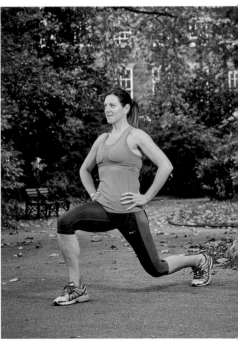

Lunge

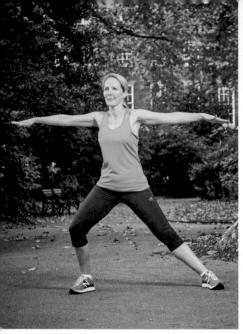
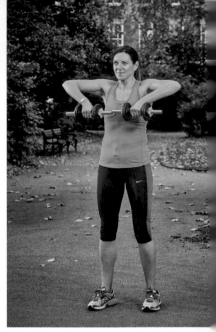

Lateral lunge

Upright row

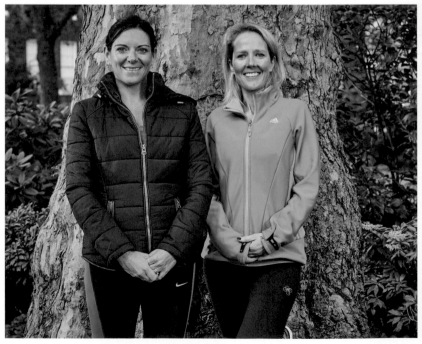

The authors: Dr Sarah Schenker and Peta Bee

WHAT TO EXPECT

You'll drop a dress size (or more): If you stick to the diet and exercise programme, you will almost certainly lose a dress size or more within the first 4–6 weeks. We have experienced it ourselves and we have seen it happen to others. If you cheat, you are only cheating yourself and the results will be slower to come.

You'll have more energy: Blood sugar levels adapt to the low GI foods you are eating and this will be followed by regulation in appetite. Foods with a low GI release their energy slowly and maintain balanced blood sugar. As you are not snacking or eating sugary foods, there are no sharp rises in your blood glucose level followed by a big dip which leaves you feeling tired and drained.

You'll burn calories at a faster rate: Because you will be exercising at a higher intensity than you are used to, results will come quickly. The workouts we've prescribed trigger your body into building more metabolically active muscle tissue and getting rid of surplus body fat. Since muscle is better at burning calories than body fat, you will become a more efficient calorie-burning machine. The result? The weight drops off and you'll look leaner in a matter of weeks.

You'll lose your sweet tooth: Incorporating fruit in meals will help you lose your sweet tooth and reduce any cravings for sugary treats. Your taste buds will get used to a subtle sweetness that the fruit can give as part of a mixed meal. You will start to look at sweets and sugary foods as a turn-off and their taste will be too intense for your muted palate.

Cravings will subside: You will start to experience the long-term satisfaction from eating well-balanced meals packed with fibre and protein. No longer will you be looking for a sweet treat to finish off a meal, or raiding the biscuit tin, half an hour after you have eaten lunch. You will also begin to adjust to feeling comfortably full rather than uncomfortable stuffed. The protein in meals helps with satiation (the point at which you feel you have eaten enough, prompting you to stop) and fibre promotes satiety, the lasting feeling of fullness that you need to observe the no snacking rule.

Skin and hair will look better: You will feel and look better as the typical problems of dry skin and brittle hair are helped by a diet full of oils, avocados, nuts and seeds. They contain vitamin E, zinc and essential fats needed for healthy looking skin, hair and nails.

You'll lose the urge to snack post-exercise: Studies have shown that higher intensity exercise suppresses appetite rather than triggers it. So, you will find that you no longer feel ravenously hungry after a workout like you did when you went for a long slow run or cycle. When volunteers have been put through gruelling HIIT workouts and then allowed to eat as much as they want at a buffet-style meal afterwards, they are surprised to find they simply can't stomach the food. It seems that pushing yourself physically even for a short time has an advantageous effect on curbing hunger hormones, eventually aiding weight loss in the long term.

You'll be less snappy: You will find that your mood settles and you suffer from fewer mood swings and better sleep as your hormones become more balanced. Our meals include foods that contain the amino acid tryptophan, which is found in turkey, oats, legumes and cottage cheese. Tryptophan helps manufacture the neurotransmitter serotonin. Serotonin helps moods and may help control sleep and appetite, which can make you feel better in yourself. Add the mood enhancing benefits of regular exercise, and friends and family will think you've been taking some happy pills.

Sarah's Top 5 Tips

- ♥ Try skipping breakfast. It won't work for everyone, but the majority of women over 35 who try it have found it makes a dramatic difference to their weight and also spurs them to eat more healthily for the rest of the day.

- ♥ Stick to one carb-based meal a day – all others should be protein and vegetable based. Government recommendations to include bread, potatoes, rice and pasta is outdated advice for life lived in a previous century.

- ♥ Never snack. You'll need to train yourself to get into this habit (and it really is a habit), but it's just a case of mind over matter. You can and will adapt if you persevere.

- ♥ Re-think the way you view food and calories. A latte with syrup, a frappucino or a muffin constitute a meal each in terms of the energy they provide and yet supply precious little in terms of valuable nutrients.

- ♥ Be creative in thought. When you think you don't have time to make a dish we've recommended, look at it from another angle – if you make 4–6 portions, you are saving 3–5 times the effort of preparing it on another occasion.

Peta's Top 5 Tips

♥ Forget about 'fuelling up' for exercise and 're-fuelling' when you finish. An entire industry of workout energy bars, drinks and snacks has arisen out of the concept that extra carbs are necessary to see you through any sort of exercise. But the concept is outdated and certainly not relevant to the kind of exercise we advocate, which lasts no longer than 45 minutes a session. Eating well and regularly will suffice.

♥ Try one session of fitness-fasting – a pre-breakfast workout – a week. Or, if you are more of an afternoon or evening exerciser, leave at least 4 hours before one weekly workout. It really helps to re-programme your body into fat-blasting mode and I personally find it invigorating.

♥ Don't carry a drink. This is a real bugbear of mine – so many people feel they can't complete a workout without constantly sipping from a water bottle. Yet there is no scientific basis for this trend whatsoever. It is almost impossible to become dehydrated when exercising for up to 45 minutes, provided you have drunk regularly beforehand. Sweat losses do not need to be replaced immediately and it is perfectly fine to top up the fluid and body salts with our delicious meals and water a couple of hours after you finish. Avoid sports drinks (highly sugared water) like the plague unless you are training for an endurance event such as a marathon.

♥ Make a pledge to yourself. Set yourself a weekly exercise goal and write it down. It might be that you aim to work out every evening as soon as you get home from work, to lift a slightly heavier weight, to meet a friend or to attempt one of the workouts. Whatever it is, the action of writing it down can have a huge impact on your chances of achieving it. I do this on a regular basis, sometimes sticking my goals to the fridge where they come under scrutiny from other members of the family. Nothing like a bit of pressure to keep you going when motivation might be running low.

♥ Prepare to adapt. There's no doubt that you will find the first few weeks of exercise fairly tough if you haven't worked out for a while. You will feel tired, stiff and sometimes a bit sore and tender. You'll sometimes wonder if it is worth carrying on. But persevere. We've designed the programme to be progressive and to allow your body time to adapt. After a month you will look back and be amazed how far you have come.

In the next chapter Sarah outlines the four-week diet plan.

CHAPTER SEVEN

THE AGELESS BODY DIET PLAN

'When you've had children, your body changes; there's history to it. I like the evolution of that history; I'm fortunate to be with somebody who likes the evolution of that history. I think it's important to not eradicate it. I look at someone's face and I see the work before I see the person.'

Cate Blanchett

Before you get started, let's just re-cap on some of the finer details of the eating plan. As you've read, we suggest a calorie intake that is significantly lower than the official recommendations for women of 40-plus, but which more than adequately meets your needs. You won't go hungry, that's for sure.

On weekdays breakfast is optional. We've provided some quick and easy recipes or options for something straightforward like multigrain toast with peanut butter for those who definitely prefer to eat something first thing, but we're convinced that, with the guilt factor alleviated, you may prefer to skip it altogether. At weekends we suggest skipping breakfast and replacing with brunch, taking no lunch and eating a more substantial supper.

Rest assured that all of your macro- and micronutrient needs are met on a daily basis. Your fats will be obtained from super-healthy sources and carbohydrates, although limited to one main serving a day, will be sustaining enough to see you through. A vast array of vegetables, fruit and grains will ensure that you don't go short on anything, and a regular intake of meat and fish will ensure your protein and iron levels are kept high.

WHAT TO AVOID:

♥ Sweetened drinks, fruit juice and smoothies, coconut water and other trendy fruit or flavoured waters (stick to eau naturel – sparkling or still)

♥ Anything that is ready-made or pre-packaged. We're aware that sometimes fruit and vegetables fit this bill, so they are excluded from the packaging rule (although it's infinitely better to get them fresh at source or from a greengrocer when you can)

♥ Diet drinks – full of nothing. A chemical concoction of no nutritional value whatsoever

♥ Snacks of any description – even the healthy pots of nuts and nibbles you can buy in wholefood stores are out

♥ Sugar-laden condiments and bottled sauces

♥ Sugary breakfast cereals – stick to the unadulterated variety if you must choose a packaged version

♥ Carbs at more than one meal a day. Don't stock up on bread, pasta and rice at every meal

♥ Processed fish and meat products

♥ Sweetened or favoured yoghurt

WHAT'S ALLOWED:

- ♥ Green tea, black coffee or water (still or sparkling) in unlimited amounts

- ♥ Red meat – once or twice a week

- ♥ Animal non-dairy protein such as chicken and fish

- ♥ Plant protein such as soya, nuts, pulses

- ♥ Dairy in the form of cheese, milk and yoghurt

- ♥ Colourful fruit and vegetables, including berries, peppers, tomatoes, melon, mango, pineapple, beetroot at every meal

- ♥ Green and white fruit and vegetables, such as green leafy veg, apples, pears, onions, cucumber, leeks at every meal

- ♥ Starchy vegetables like potatoes, sweet potato, root veg, squashes, peas, corn

- ♥ Whole grains – brown rice, quinoa

- ♥ Healthy fats from avocados, nuts, oils, oily fish

WEEK 1

	Breakfast	Lunch	Dinner
Monday	Oat berry smoothie	Oatcakes with cottage cheese mixed with pear and walnuts	Grilled seabass 1 sweet potato (cut into wedges and oven baked) ½ head of broccoli
Tuesday	Wholegrain sourdough toast with a poached egg ½ grapefruit mixed with Greek yoghurt	Curried carrot and chickpea soup (with a toasted wholemeal pitta if no breakfast)	Chicken, butternut squash and baby sweetcorn stir fry
Wednesday	Pot of yoghurt with banana, berries and chopped nuts	Chicken, avocado, apple and hazelnut salad	Lemony prawns with white beans
Thursday	1 slice of sourdough toast 1 boiled or poached egg (or peanut butter) ½ grapefruit and Greek yoghurt	Curried carrot and chickpea soup	Apple and pork meatballs in a spicy tomato sauce
Friday	Berry porridge	Crab and avocado lettuce wrap	Halloumi kebabs with watermelon and feta salad
Saturday	Buckwheat pancakes with cherries		Lamb tagine with jewelled quinoa
Sunday	Skinny mackerel kedgeree		Turkey mince and kidney bean chilli

WEEK 2

	Breakfast	Lunch	Dinner
Monday	Oat berry smoothie	Wholemeal pitta pocket with hummus, grated carrot, red pepper strips and baby spinach leaves	Grilled salmon with sweet potato mash and broccoli
Tuesday	Wholegrain sourdough toast with a poached egg ½ grapefruit mixed with Greek yoghurt	Kale and red lentil soup (add toasted sourdough bread with cheese if no breakfast)	Tofu stir fry
Wednesday	Pot of yoghurt with banana, berries and chopped nuts	Butternut squash and chickpea salad	Tuna steak with spicy mango salsa
Thursday	1 slice of sourdough toast 1 boiled or poached egg (or peanut butter) ½ grapefruit and Greek yoghurt	Kale and red lentil soup	Spicy chicken and radish salad
Friday	Berry porridge	Brazil nut dip with oatcakes and veg sticks	Turkey and apricot meatballs with bulgur wheat
Saturday	Spicy eggs		Beef and Jerusalem artichoke stew
Sunday	Date and rice porridge		Lime and coriander chicken with Puy lentils

WEEK 3

	Breakfast	Lunch	Dinner
Monday	Oat berry smoothie	Crushed new potatoes with mackerel and mushrooms	Baked pistachio chicken with sugar snap peas
Tuesday	Wholegrain sourdough toast with a poached egg ½ grapefruit mixed with Greek yoghurt	Spicy sweetcorn chowder	Pork stir fry
Wednesday	Pot of yoghurt with banana, berries and chopped nuts	Beetroot, feta and orange salad	Crab cakes
Thursday	1 slice of sourdough toast 1 boiled or poached egg (or peanut butter) ½ grapefruit and Greek yoghurt	Spicy sweetcorn chowder	Turkey mince and kidney bean chilli
Friday	Berry porridge	Nut and bean tabbouleh	French fish stew
Saturday	Pepper frittata		Lamb with barley
Sunday	Avocado hash		Citrus salmon

WEEK 4

	Breakfast	Lunch	Dinner
Monday	Oat berry smoothie	Avocado and hummus wrap	Grilled sardines with salsa verde
Tuesday	Wholegrain sourdough toast with a poached egg ½ grapefruit mixed with Greek yoghurt	Prawn pho	Tofu stir fry
Wednesday	Pot of yoghurt with banana, berries and chopped nuts	Minted pea dip with oatcakes and veg sticks	Chicken soba noodles
Thursday	1 slice of sourdough toast 1 boiled or poached egg (or peanut butter) ½ grapefruit and Greek yoghurt	Prawn pho	Turkey mince and kidney bean chilli
Friday	Berry porridge	Chicken and butter bean salad	French fish stew
Saturday	Grilled fruit with nuts and yoghurt		Lamb tagine with jewelled quinoa
Sunday	Muffin stack		Beef and Jerusalem artichoke stew

CHAPTER EIGHT

RECIPES AND SHOPPING LISTS

WEEK 1

Oat berry smoothie

Serves 1
  small banana, roughly chopped
  ½ punnet of berries
  50ml/2fl oz milk or almond milk
  2 tbsp Greek yoghurt
  1 tbsp oats

In a blender, whizz together the fruit, milk and yoghurt. Stir in the oats and pour into a flask. Keep chilled in the fridge until ready to eat or take with you to work.

Berry porridge

Serves 1

  4 tbsp porridge oats
  200ml/7fl oz milk or almond milk
  ½ tsp mixed spice
  1 tbsp sunflower seeds
  ½ punnet of berries

Cook the oats in the milk and when creamy, stir in the berries, mixed spice and seeds.

Buckwheat pancakes with cherries

Serves 2

  250g/9oz cherries, stoned and halved
  250ml/10fl oz Greek yoghurt
  100g/4oz buckwheat flour
  2 tbsp self-raising flour
  1 tsp cinnamon
  1 tsp bicarbonate of soda
  2 eggs
  150ml/5fl oz buttermilk
  2 tbsp honey (optional)
  few knobs of butter

Mix the cherries into the Greek yoghurt. Mix the flours, cinnamon and bicarb in a large bowl. Make a well in the centre and crack in the eggs. Gradually whisk in with the buttermilk to make a smooth batter and then stir in the honey to your desired level of sweetness. You may want to use less or none at all.

Melt a knob of butter in a non-stick frying pan. Add spoonfuls of batter to make pancakes about 8–10cm across. Cook for a couple of minutes until set on the bottom and bubbles appear on the surface, then flip and cook the other side. Keep the pancakes warm in the oven on a low heat while you finish up the batter. Serve the pancakes with a dollop of the yogurt and cherry mixture.

Smoked mackerel and rice (kedgeree)

Serves 2
  140g/4oz brown basmati rice
  2 eggs
  1 tbsp olive oil
  4 spring onions
  1 red chilli, deseeded and chopped
  2 tbsp medium curry powder
  1 tsp mustard seeds
  1 tsp cayenne pepper
  2 smoked mackerel fillets, flaked
  handful of flat-leaf parsley, chopped
  salt and freshly ground black pepper

Put the rice into a pan with 280ml/10fl oz of cold water and a pinch of salt. Bring to the boil, stir, cover and reduce the heat. Simmer gently for 15–20 minutes, or until all the liquid has been absorbed.

Boil the eggs in a separate pan for 7 minutes.

Meanwhile, heat the oil in a non-stick frying pan over a medium heat and soften the onion and chilli for 5 minutes. Add all the spices and fry for a further 1–2 minutes.

Drain the rice and stir into the spicy onion with a splash of water and the mackerel. Season with black pepper, then heat through gently for a few minutes until piping hot.

Peel and quarter the boiled eggs. Stir parsley into the rice, divide between two bowls and top with the egg quarters.

Curried carrot and chickpea soup

Serves 2

   Olive oil
   1 red onion, chopped
   2 stalks of celery, chopped
   1 knob of ginger, peeled and grated
   2 tsp garam masala
   6 carrots, peeled and chopped
   2 parsnips, peeled and chopped
   1 litre/1 ¾ pint of vegetable stock
   1 tin of chickpeas/garbanzo beans, rinsed

Heat a drizzle of olive oil in a large pan, add the onion, celery, ginger and garam masala and cook for 5 minutes until softened. Add the carrots, parsnips and stock, season well and bring to the boil. Allow to simmer for 25 minutes and then allow to cool. Tip into a blender and whizz until smooth. Return to the pan and add the chickpeas/garbanzo beans, reheat and simmer for 10 minutes. (The rest will keep in the fridge for 2–3 days).

Chicken, avocado, apple and hazelnut salad

Serves 1
    1 chicken breast, grilled
    ½ bag of mixed leaves
    ¼ cucumber, chopped
    ½ ripe avocado, sliced
    1 spring onion, sliced
    1 small apple, cored and thinly sliced
    1 tbsp hazelnuts
    handful each of basil and mint leaves
    dash of balsamic vinegar
    dash of extra virgin olive oil
    freshly ground black pepper

Simply mix all the salad ingredients together in a small salad bowl, season with freshly ground black pepper and serve with the chicken breast.

Crab and avocado lettuce wrap

Serves 1
    1 baby gem lettuce
    100g/4oz white crab meat
    ½ an avocado, chopped
    1 tbsp crème fraiche
    1 tsp Dijon mustard
    squeeze of lemon juice
    small handful of chopped dill
    1 tsp capers

Separate the leaves of a gem lettuce.

Place the crab meat with the chopped avocado in a bowl. Mix the crème fraiche and Dijon mustard, lemon juice, chopped dill and capers. Toss the crab and avocado in the dressing and scoop up with the leaves.

Chicken, butternut squash and baby corn stir fry

Serves 1

½ butternut squash
drizzle of olive oil
drizzle of rapeseed oil
1 chicken fillet, sliced
1 clove garlic, crushed
small piece of grated ginger
2 spring onions, sliced
100g/4oz mangetout/snow peas
½ red pepper (cut into strips)
100g/4oz baby corn
1 tbsp soy sauce
1 tbsp balsamic vinegar
drizzle of honey

Preheat the oven to 180°C/350°F/Gas mark 5. Place the butternut squash on a baking tray, cut side up. Drizzle with olive oil, season with salt and pepper and bake in the oven for 20 minutes. Remove from the oven and allow to cool until you can handle it. Peel away the skin and thickly slice.

Heat the rapeseed oil in a wok, add the chicken, garlic and ginger and cook for about 5 minutes. Then add the other vegetables and cook for a further 2 minutes. Finally add the soy sauce, vinegar and honey and cook for another 2 minutes.

Lemony prawns with white beans

Serves 2

  2 leeks, thickly sliced
  knob of fresh ginger, peeled and grated
  ½ red chilli, chopped
  1 clove garlic, crushed
  juice of 1 lemon
  2 tbsp olive oil
  200g/7oz raw prawns
  ½ x 400g/14oz tin cannellini beans, rinsed and drained
  2 handfuls of fresh coriander/cilantro, chopped
  salt and freshly ground black pepper

Put the leeks in a steamer and cook for 4–5 minutes until tender. Set aside.

  Using a small grinder, processor or pestle and mortar, make a paste with the ginger, chilli, garlic and lemon juice. Heat the olive oil in a pan over a medium heat, tip in the paste and sauté for a couple of minutes.

  Add the prawns and beans and cook for 10 minutes until the prawns are pink and cooked through. Add the leeks to the pan and mix through. Season with salt and pepper to taste and then scatter with the chopped coriander/cilantro before serving.

Apple and pork meatballs in a spicy tomato sauce

Serves 2

- 2 oatcakes
- 1 large shallot, roughly chopped
- 1 apple, peeled, cored and roughly chopped
- 1 tbsp chopped fresh lemon thyme leaves
- 300g/11oz lean pork mince
- 2 tbsp olive oil
- 1 medium red onion, chopped
- 1 clove garlic, peeled and chopped
- ½ red pepper, chopped
- handful of fresh basil, stalks chopped and leaves torn
- chilli flakes to taste
- 400g/14oz tin chopped tomatoes
- 100g/4oz fresh tomatoes, skinned and deseeded, roughly chopped
- 1 tsp tomato purée
- dash of Worcestershire sauce
- 150g/5oz green beans

Place the oatcakes, shallot, apple and lemon thyme in a food processor and whizz until finely chopped. Place the pork mince in a large bowl and season with salt and pepper. Add the oat and apple mix and stir well to combine and then shape the mixture into 10–12 small balls, using damp hands so that the mixture doesn't stick.

Heat the olive oil in a large non-stick frying pan and brown the meatballs over a medium heat for 4–5 minutes, turning occasionally to colour evenly. Remove from the pan and drain on kitchen paper.

For the sauce, use the same pan to fry the onion, garlic, pepper and basil stalks for about 8–10 minutes until softened. Add the chilli flakes and cook for a further 2–3 minutes. Add the tomatoes, tinned and fresh, purée and add a splash of water, if needed, plus the Worcestershire sauce to taste. Simmer for 5 minutes and then add meatballs and basil leaves, cover and simmer for 20 minutes. Serve with the steamed green beans.

Halloumi kebabs with watermelon and feta salad

Serves 2

pinch of chilli flakes
handful of coriander/cilantro, chopped
squeeze of lemon juice
drizzle of olive oil
1 courgette/zucchini, cut into chunks
1 red pepper, diced
100g/4oz pack halloumi cheese, cubed
1 small red onion, diced
200g/7oz watermelon, seeds removed and diced
50g/2oz feta cheese, diced
handful of fresh flat-leaf parsley, chopped
handful of fresh mint, chopped
25g/1oz pitted black olives, halved
2 tbsp olive oil
juice of a lime
freshly ground black pepper

Mix the chilli, coriander/cilantro, lemon juice, oil, courgette/zucchini, pepper and halloumi. Leave to marinate for 30 minutes.

Soak two wooden skewers for 20 minutes. Thread the veg and halloumi onto the skewers. Cook under a grill, for 7–8 minutes, turning halfway through and basting with the remaining marinade.

Meanwhile make the salad by combining all the remaining ingredients in a large bowl, season with black pepper and dress with the lime juice and olive oil.

Lamb tagine with jewelled quinoa

Serves 4

2 tbsp oil
1 onion, finely chopped
2 cloves garlic, finely chopped
1 tsp ground coriander/cilantro
1 tbsp ras el hanout
400g/14oz boneless lamb from the leg, trimmed and cubed
200g/7oz butternut squash, peeled and diced
400g/14oz tin chickpeas/garbanzo beans, rinsed and drained
200g/7oz soft dried apricots
400g/14oz tin chopped tomatoes
500ml/1 pint lamb or beef stock
200g/7oz quinoa
50g/2oz pomegranate seeds
50g/2oz flaked almonds
zest of 1 lemon
small bunch fresh coriander/cilantro, roughly chopped

Preheat the oven to 200°C/400°F/Gas mark 6. Heat the oil in a flameproof casserole dish, add the onion and cook for 5 minutes over a medium heat until softened. Add the garlic, ground coriander/cilantro and ras el hanout and cook, stirring, for a couple of minutes more.

Add the cubed lamb, butternut squash, chickpeas/garbanzo beans and apricots to the casserole, then pour over the tomatoes and stock. Season well with salt and pepper and bring to the boil. Put the lid on and transfer to the oven. After 1 hour, turn down the oven to 150°C/300°F/Gas mark 4, stir the tagine and return to the oven, uncovered, for a further 30 minutes.

Prepare the quinoa according to the packet instructions. Stir in the pomegranate and almonds and then sprinkle over the lemon zest and chopped coriander/cilantro. Serve with the lamb.

Turkey mince and kidney bean chilli

Serves 4

   drizzle of olive oil
   ½–1 tsp chilli flakes
   1 tsp cumin
   1 onion, finely diced
   400g/14oz turkey mince
   200g/7oz mushrooms, diced
   1 red pepper, deseeded and diced
   2 x 400g/14oz tins choppped tomatoes
   1 tbsp tomato purée
   1 cinnamon stick, snapped in half
   400g/14oz tin red kidney beans, drained and rinsed

Heat the oil in a large pan and add the chilli flakes, cumin and onion and cook over a medium heat for 8–10 minutes until softened. Add the mince and continue to cook for 2–3 minutes and then add the mushrooms and pepper and cook for a further 2–3 minutes. Add the tomatoes, tomato purée and the cinnamon stick, stir thoroughly and keep over a medium heat for 20 minutes. Add the kidney beans and cook for a further 5–10 minutes. Serve with a green salad.

Shopping list
  2 bananas
  1 punnet of berries
  2 pints of milk (or 1 pint and 1 carton of almond milk)
  1 large tub of Greek yogurt
  1 punnet of cherries
  6 eggs
  1 carton of buttermilk
  Bunch of spring onions
  1 red chilli
  2 fillets of smoked mackerel
  Bunch each of parsley, coriander/cilantro, thyme, mint, basil, dill
  4 red onions
  2 stalks of celery
  Knob of ginger
  6 carrots
  2 parsnips
  2 chicken breasts
  1 bag of mixed leaves
  1 cucumber
  1 avocado
  2 apples
  1 butternut squash
  1 pack of mangetout/snow peas and baby corn
  3 red peppers
  Head of garlic

2 leeks
1 lemon
1 bag of shallots
200g/7oz prawns
300g/11oz minced pork
4 tomatoes
1 pack of green beans
1 courgette/zucchini
1 pack of halloumi
Half a watermelon
1 pack of feta
1 lime
1 pomegranate
400g/14oz turkey mince
400g/14oz boneless lamb leg
1 punnet of mushrooms
1 grapefruit
1 tub of cottage cheese
1 tub of crème fraiche
1 pear
1 Gem lettuce
1 seabass
1 sweet potato
1 head of broccoli

Store cupboard
1 tin of crab
Jar of olives
Jar of capers
Sunflower seeds
Hazelnuts
Oats

Oatcakes
Almonds
Walnuts
Dried apricots
Honey
Buckwheat flour
Brown basmati rice
Quinoa
Olive oil
Stock
2 tins of chickpeas/garbanzo beans
1 small tin of cannellini beans
1 tin of kidney beans
4 tins of tomatoes
Worcestershire sauce
Soy sauce
Tomato purée
Balsamic vinegar
Dijon mustard
Spices – cayenne, chilli flakes, cumin seeds, coriander/cilantro, cinnamon, mustard seeds, curry powder, garam masala, ras el hanout

WEEK 2

Spicy eggs

Serves 2
2 tbsp olive oil
½ onion, diced

½ fresh red chilli, deseeded and chopped
1 clove garlic, crushed
1 red pepper, deseeded and roughly chopped
400g/14oz tin chopped tomatoes
1 tbsp tomato purée
½ tsp hot paprika
pinch of cayenne pepper
2 large eggs
1 tbsp chopped fresh parsley
salt and black pepper

Heat the olive oil in a large frying pan. Add the onion and chilli and sauté for a few minutes until the onion begins to soften. Add the garlic and red pepper and cook for 5 minutes over a medium heat until softened.

Stir in the tomatoes and then add the tomato purée, paprika and cayenne pepper. Reduce the heat and simmer for a further 10 minutes until the liquid starts to reduce.

Season with the salt and plenty of black pepper, then crack the eggs directly into the tomato mixture. Cover and cook for 10 minutes, or until the egg whites are firm, the yolks still runny and the sauce has reduced slightly. Garnish with the chopped parsley and serve immediately.

Date and rice porridge

Serves 2
200g/7oz cooked brown basmati rice
250ml/10fl oz milk
½ tsp mixed spice

drizzle of honey
1 small egg
1 tbsp pumpkin seeds
6 chopped dates

Combine the cooked brown rice, milk, spice and honey in a small saucepan. Bring to the boil, then reduce heat to low and simmer for 20 minutes.

Beat the egg in a small bowl. Temper the egg by whisking in some of the hot rice, a tablespoon at a time until you have incorporated about 6 tablespoons. Stir the egg into the rice along with the seeds and continue cooking over low heat for 1–2 minutes to thicken. Stir in the chopped dates just before serving.

Kale and red lentil soup

Serves 2
olive oil
pinch of chilli flakes
1 red onion, chopped
½ leek, chopped
2 stalks of celery, chopped
1 head of kale, shredded
1 litre/1 ¾ pint of vegetable stock
50g/2oz dried red lentils

Heat a drizzle of olive oil in a pan and add the chilli flakes, onion, leek and celery and cook for 5 minutes until softened. Add the kale, stock and lentils, season well and bring to the boil, and then allow to simmer for 25 minutes.

Butternut squash and chickpea salad

Serves 2

1 large sweet potato, peeled and diced

½ butternut squash, peeled and diced (you can buy a bag
of sweet potato and butternut squash ready diced)

½ x 400g/14oz tin chickpeas/garbanzo beans, drained and rinsed

25g/1oz unskinned hazelnuts

2 handfuls of watercress leaves

12 cherry tomatoes, halved

2 spring onions, chopped

½ cucumber, chopped

2 tbsp olive oil

2 tbsp balsamic vinegar

Preheat the oven to 190°C/375°F/Gas mark 5. Place the sweet potato and butternut squash in a pan, cover with boiling water and simmer for 5–6 minutes until tender. Drain well and then spread out on a baking sheet. Drizzle with half the olive oil and bake in the oven for 15 minutes until golden.

Transfer the baked sweet potato and butternut squash to a large bowl and add the chickpeas, hazelnuts, watercress, tomatoes, spring onions and cucumber. Toss together and dress with the remaining olive oil and balsamic vinegar.

Brazil nut dip

Makes 3–4 portions, can be kept in the fridge for 2–3 days

150g/5oz Brazil nuts, soaked in water for 24 hours, drained
and rinsed

2–3 cloves garlic
3 tbsp lemon juice
2 tbsp rapeseed oil
2 tbsp tahini
pinch of cayenne pepper
sea salt and freshly ground pepper

Place all the ingredients into a food processor and blend until you have a smooth paste. Add a little water to loosen if necessary. Taste and adjust the seasoning and then transfer to a bowl. Cover with cling film and chill in the fridge until ready to serve.

Tofu stir fry

Serves 2

25g/1oz unsalted cashew nuts
1 tbsp rapeseed oil
1 head of broccoli, cut into small florets
2 cloves garlic, sliced
1 red chilli, deseeded and finely sliced
1 bunch spring onions, sliced
100g/4oz frozen soya beans
2 heads of pak choi, quartered
200g/7oz marinated tofu pieces
1 tbsp hoisin sauce
1 tbsp soy sauce

Dry fry the cashew nuts in a small pan for 1–2 minutes. Be careful not to let them catch, they burn very easily.

Heat the oil in a non-stick wok over a high heat. Add the broccoli, then fry for 5 minutes or until just tender, adding a splash of water if it begins to catch. Add the garlic and chilli and fry for 1 minute before adding the spring onions, soya beans, pak choi and tofu pieces. Stir-fry for 2–3 minutes and then add the hoisin and soy sauces and toasted cashews. Stir to warm through before serving.

Tuna steak with spicy mango salsa

Serves 2

  1 tbsp olive oil
  zest and juice of 2 limes
  1 red chilli, finely sliced
  1 clove garlic, crushed
  2 tuna steaks
  1 mango, diced
  1 red onion, finely sliced
  200g/7oz green beans
  handful each of watercress and spinach leaves
  handful of fresh coriander/cilantro, chopped

Mix the oil with the lime zest, half the juice, chilli and garlic. Place the tuna steaks in a dish, coat thoroughly with the chilli mixture and allow to marinate for at least 30 minutes (preferably overnight).

Place the mango pieces in a large bowl, add the remaining lime juice and the red onion. Cook the tuna on a hot griddle pan for 5 minutes each side.

Meanwhile, blanch the green beans for 1 minute in boiling water, drain, run under cold water and then add to the mango with the leaves and coriander/cilantro. Toss together, season and serve with the tuna.

Spicy chicken and radish salad

Serves 1

  1 chicken breast
  drizzle of olive oil
  pinch each of chilli flakes and cumin seeds
  handful each of spinach and watercress leaves
  handful each of parsley, coriander/cilantro and mint leaves,
  chopped
  2 spring onions
  5 radishes, quartered
  1 tbsp hazelnuts
  2 tbsp Greek yogurt
  1 tbsp crème fraiche
  juice from half a lemon

Preheat the oven to 190°C/370°F/Gas mark 5. Drizzle the chicken breast with oil, season with a pinch of salt and plenty of black pepper and sprinkle with the chilli flakes and cumin seeds. Bake in the oven for 20 minutes.

Meanwhile arrange the leaves, herbs, spring onions and radishes in a bowl and throw in the hazelnuts. Make a dressing by mixing the yogurt and crème fraiche together, stir in the lemon juice and season well.

Remove the chicken from the oven, allow to cool slightly and then shred into the leaves. Add the dressing and gently toss together.

Turkey and apricot meatballs with bulgur wheat

Serves 2

  80g/3oz bulgur wheat
  For the meatballs:

250g/9oz turkey mince
½ onion, finely chopped
6 dried apricots, finely chopped
50g/2oz oatcakes, crumbled
1 tbsp flat-leaf parsley, finely chopped
1 tsp baharat spice mix
1 small egg, beaten
1 tbsp olive oil
3 spring onions, chopped
50g/2oz blanched almonds
50g/2oz pomegranate seeds
100g/4oz cherry tomatoes, diced
squeeze of lemon juice

Cook the bulgur wheat according to the packet instructions.

Place all the ingredients for the meatballs into a bowl, season with a pinch of salt and plenty of black pepper and mix together with your hands to form into evenly sized small balls.

Heat the oil in a frying pan and over a high heat sear half the meatballs for 5 minutes until browned, then turn down the heat and cook for another 10 minutes until cooked through. Remove the meatballs and keep warm.

Using the same pan add the spring onions and cook for 3 minutes.

Place the bulgur wheat in a bowl and stir in the spring onions. Add the almonds, pomegranate and tomatoes and squeeze over some lemon juice, and then serve with the meatballs.

Beef and Jerusalem artichoke stew

Serves 4 (or half can be frozen)
  2 tbsp olive oil
  900g/2lb lean beef steak, diced
  flour, for dusting
  6 shallots, quartered
  3 large carrots, diced
  3 Jerusalem artichokes, peeled and diced
  3 parsnips, diced
  ½ butternut squash, diced
  handful of fresh sage
  400g/14oz tin black-eyed beans
  500ml/1 pint red wine
  300ml/10fl oz beef stock
  2 tbsp tomato purée
  salt and freshly ground black pepper

Preheat the oven to 150°C/300°F/Gas mark 2. Heat the oil in a large casserole dish. Toss the meat in the flour and place in the casserole dish with the vegetables. Add all the other ingredients, cover with a lid and cook in the oven for 3–4 hours.

Lime and coriander chicken with Puy lentils

Serves 2
  2 skinless chicken fillets
  drizzle of olive oil
  ½ cucumber, sliced lengthways, deseeded and cut into
    crescents

handful of coriander/cilantro, including finely chopped stalks
handful of mint leaves
1 tsp of Chinese five-spice
1 tbsp Thai fish sauce
1 tsp sesame oil
1 spring onion, finely sliced diagonally
2 tbsp lime juice
lime wedges to serve
1 tsp rapeseed oil
1 clove garlic, finely chopped
½ red pepper, finely chopped
1 shallot, finely chopped
300g/10oz Puy lentils
150ml/5fl oz white wine
300ml/10fl oz hot chicken stock
handful of rocket

Preheat oven to 190°C/370°F/Gas mark 6. Drizzle the olive oil over the chicken breast and then season with salt and pepper. Bake, covered, in oven for 20 minutes until cooked through and juices run clear. Allow to cool. Tear chicken into shreds and place in a bowl with the cucumber, most of the coriander and mint. Make a dressing from the five-spice, fish sauce, sesame oil, spring onion, lime juice, and season. Combine with the chicken mixture and set aside.

To make the Puy lentils, heat the rapeseed oil in a frying pan over a medium heat. Add the garlic, pepper and shallot and fry until soft. Add the lentils, stir well and continue cooking for one minute.

Increase the heat and add the wine. Boil the liquid to reduce by half, then add the stock and reduce the heat to simmer for

15 minutes, until the lentils are cooked through. Season with salt and freshly ground black pepper.

Place a pile of the lentils into the middle of a plate and top with the chicken and serve with a handful of rocket and a sprinkling of coriander/cilantro leaves.

Shopping list
  2 pints of milk/almond milk (or 1 of each)
  Large pot of Greek yogurt
  1 punnet of berries
  2 bananas
  6 eggs
  1 grapefruit
  Pack of wholemeal pittas
  1 tub of hummus
  5 carrots
  3 red peppers
  1 bag of spinach leaves
  2 red onions
  2 red chillies
  1 lime
  1 lemon
  1 mango
  Bunch of spring onions
  Bunch each of fresh herbs – parsley, sage, coriander/cilantro, mint
  1 leek
  1 bag of kale
  2 sweet pototoes
  1 butternut squash
  1 bag of watercress

1 pack of pak choi
1 bag of radishes
1 pack of tofu
1 pomegranate
250g/9oz turkey mince
3 parsnips
1 Jerusalem artichoke
2 chicken breasts
1 salmon steak
1 tuna steak
900g/2lb beef stewing steak

Leftover from last week
Garlic
Shallots
Tomatoes
Cucumber
Broccoli
Green beans
Celery
Crème fraiche

Store cupboard
Dates
Pumpkin seeds
Red lentils
1 tin of chickpeas/garbanzo beans
1 tin of black-eyed beans
1 tin of Puy lentils
Brazil nuts
Cashew nuts
Tahini paste

Rapeseed oil
Sesame oil
1 bag of frozen soya beans
Hoisin sauce
Thai fish sauce
Bulgur wheat
Spices – Chinese five-spice
Red and white wine

WEEK 3

Pepper frittata

Serves 2
2 red peppers
1 tbsp olive oil
1 small onion, chopped
2 cloves garlic, crushed
75g/3oz chorizo, skinned or ½ x 400g tin chickpeas/garbanzo beans, drained
1 tsp smoked paprika
100g/4oz spinach leaves
4 large eggs, beaten
salt and freshly ground black pepper

Preheat the oven to 180°C/350°F/Gas mark 5. Place the peppers on a baking sheet, cut side down, and bake in the oven for 15 minutes until the skin has blistered. Remove from the oven and allow to cool. When cool enough to handle, remove the skins and roughly chop the flesh.

Heat the olive oil in a large frying pan over a medium heat and sauté the onion and garlic until soft. Dice the chorizo, if using, and add to the pan, or add the chickpeas/garbanzo beans, and paprika. Sauté everything together for about 5 minutes.

Add the spinach and keep stirring until it wilts and everything starts to meld together in the pan. Add the eggs and seasoning and stir gently to incorporate the eggs into the whole mixture, then allow to set over a medium heat – this should take about 2 minutes.

Preheat the grill to hot, then slide the whole pan under the grill to set the top of the frittata. It will only take a minute or two to become light golden and puffed up.

Avocado hash

Serves 2

200g/7oz new or waxy potatoes, cut into cubes
1 red chilli, slit lengthways and deseeded
2 tbsp rapeseed oil
1 clove garlic, chopped
1 tsp Cajun seasoning
200g/7oz tin baby corn, drained and rinsed
200g/7oz tin black beans, drained and rinsed
2 eggs
1 ripe avocado, chopped
lime wedges
salt and freshly ground black pepper

Cook the potatoes in a pan of boiling salted water for 5 minutes. Drain and allow to steam dry. Slice half the chilli into strips and set aside; finely chop the other half.

Heat half the rapeseed oil in a pan over a medium heat and fry the potatoes for about 10–15 minutes until golden. Add the chopped chilli, garlic, Cajun seasoning, sweetcorn and black beans and heat through for about 5 minutes; season to taste. Keep warm while you fry the eggs.

Heat the remaining oil in a frying pan and fry the eggs until cooked to your liking. Divide the potatoes between two bowls and top each one with a fried egg, some chopped avocado and the sliced chilli. Serve with the lime wedges.

Crushed new potatoes with mackerel and mushrooms

Serves 1

150g/5oz new potatoes
1 smoked mackerel fillet
1 tbsp crème fraiche
1–2 tsp hot horseradish sauce (or a knob of grated fresh horseradish)
small handful of chives, snipped
squeeze of lemon juice
2 handfuls of watercress
2 spring onions, chopped

Place the potatoes in a large pan of water, bring to the boil and allow to simmer for 15 minutes until tender. Drain and allow to cool and then lightly crush with the back of a spoon. Remove the skin from the mackerel and flake the flesh.

Mix together the crème fraiche, horseradish, chives, lemon juice and season with plenty of black pepper.

Place the watercress in a bowl (or lunchbox), add the spring onions, potatoes and the fish. Add the dressing and gently toss together.

Spicy sweetcorn chowder

Serves 2

   1 tbsp olive oil
   1 leek, finely sliced
   2 stalks of celery, finely sliced
   300g/10oz celeriac, peeled and cut into small cubes
   1 litre fish stock
   zest of 1 lemon
   2 tbsp Greek yogurt
   ½ or 1 red chilli, finely sliced
   330g/12oz tin baby corn, rinsed and drained
   250g/9oz skinless and boneless white fish, cut into chunks
   handful of chives, snipped

Heat the oil in a large pan over a medium heat, tip in the leeks and celery and fry gently for 5 minutes until softened, but not coloured. Add the celeriac and cook for a further minute. Add the stock and lemon zest, cover and simmer for 12–15 minutes or until the celeriac is tender. Using a slotted spoon, remove half the celeriac and leeks from the stock and set aside.

Transfer the remaining celeriac, leeks and stock to a blender or food processor and whizz until smooth; stir in the yogurt. Return to the pan and add the baby corn, fish and reserved celeriac and leeks. Cover and gently heat for 3–4 minutes until the fish is just cooked through – take care not to boil. Stir in the chives and add seasoning to taste.

Beetroot, feta and orange salad

Serves 1

1 small golden beetroot
½ orange
1 pink apple, cored and quartered
½ head of chicory
2 spring onions, sliced diagonally
40g/1 ½oz feta, crumbled
handful of walnut halves
For the dressing:
1 tbsp red wine vinegar
zest and juice of remaining ½ orange
1 tbsp olive oil
pinch of salt and freshly ground black pepper

Preheat the oven to 200°C/400°F/Gas mark 6. Put the beetroot in a roasting tin with a couple of centimetres of water in the bottom. Cover with foil and roast in the oven for 30 minutes. (If making for lunch, do this the night before.)

Meanwhile put all the dressing ingredients into a screw-top jar and shake until well combined.

Remove the beetroot from the oven and when it is cool enough to handle, peel off the skin, top and tail it and slice into rounds. Toss in a little of the dressing.

Use a sharp knife to trim the skin and pith of the orange and chop the segments. Cut the apple quarters into thin slices. Trim the head of chicory and separate the leaves, discarding the outer leaves.

Arrange the chicory leaves in a bowl (or lunchbox) and then add the sliced beetroot, orange, apple and spring onion. Crumble the feta on top, add the walnuts and drizzle with the remaining dressing.

Nut and bean tabbouleh

Serves 1

- 30g/1oz bulgur wheat
- handful of fresh flat-leaf parsley, finely chopped
- handful of fresh mint, leaves finely chopped
- ½ small red onion, peeled and finely chopped
- 1 tomato, chopped
- handful of hazelnuts
- 2 tbsp tinned haricot beans/navy beans, drained and rinsed
- juice of ½ lemon
- 1 tbsp olive oil
- salt and freshly ground black pepper

Place the bulgur wheat in a small bowl (or lunchbox) and cover with 60ml boiling water. Stir, then set aside for 20 minutes, or until the bulgur wheat has absorbed all of the water. Then fluff it with a fork until the grains are separated. Add the parsley, mint and red onion to the tomato and mix until well combined, then stir in the hazelnuts and haricot/navy beans.

Drizzle over the lemon juice and olive oil and add seasoning to taste.

Baked pistachio chicken with sugar snap peas

Serves 1

  2 chicken drumsticks, skin removed
  juice of ½ lemon
  1 tbsp wholemeal flour
  1 tsp curry powder
  handful of pistachios
  handful of coriander/cilantro leaves, roughly torn
  pinch of cayenne pepper
  1 tbsp rapeseed oil
  1 egg, beaten
  salt and freshly ground black pepper

Preheat the oven to 220°C/430°F/Gas mark 7.

Squeeze the lemon juice over the chicken drumsticks. Mix the flour, curry powder and seasoning together in a shallow dish. Toss the drumsticks in the flour mixture until well coated on all sides. Tap off the surplus flour and arrange the drumsticks on a plate, reserving the unused flour.

Put the pistachios, coriander leaves/cilantro, reserved flour and cayenne pepper into a food processor and pulse until well combined. Tip out onto a shallow plate.

Pour the oil into a roasting tin and swirl to coat the bottom of the tin with the oil. Put the empty tin in the oven while you coat the chicken.

Dip each drumstick into the beaten egg and then into the pistachio mixture. Add the drumsticks to the hot roasting tin, turning to coat in the oil, and cook in the oven for 15 minutes. Pour off any excess oil and return to the oven for a further 5 minutes to get really crisp. Drain on kitchen paper and serve with some steamed sugar snap peas.

Pork stir fry

Serves 1

    spray of olive oil
    1 pork fillet, thinly sliced
    100g/4oz tenderstem broccoli, chopped
    small tin water chestnuts, diced
    1 red pepper, de-seeded and sliced
    2 spring onions, sliced
    1 tbsp soy sauce

Heat the oil in a wok. Add the pork and cook for 2–3 minutes. Add the remaining ingredients and sauté for another five minutes. Transfer to a dish and serve warm.

Crab cakes

Serves 2

    1 large sweet potato, peeled and diced
    250g/9oz crabmeat
    pinch of cayenne pepper
    1 tbsp wholegrain mustard
    splash of Worcestershire sauce
    4 spring onions, chopped
    handful of parsley, chopped
    juice of half a lemon
    freshly ground black pepper
    flour for dusting

Add the sweet potato to a pan of boiling water and boil for 10 minutes until soft, drain well and allow to steam for a minute and then place in a bowl and mash with a fork or potato masher. Mix in the crabmeat, cayenne pepper, mustard, Worcestershire sauce, spring onions and parsley. Season and stir in the lemon juice. Place the bowl in the fridge for a few hours. Sprinkle some flour on a clean surface and your hands and shape the mixture into 4 patties. Heat a little oil in a non-stick frying pan and when hot, fry the crab cakes for 3 minutes on each side. Serve with salad.

French fish stew

Serves 2
    drizzle of olive oil
    1 shallot, peeled and finely chopped
    1 bulb fennel, finely chopped
    1 clove garlic, peeled and finely chopped
    splash of vermouth or dry white wine
    300ml/10fl oz chicken stock
    ½ tin chopped tomatoes
    250g/9oz mixed seafood
    100g/4oz spinach

Heat the oil in a large pan, add the shallot, fennel and garlic and cook for 5 minutes until softened. Add the vermouth/wine and let bubble for a minute. Pour in the chicken stock and tomatoes and bring to the boil. Simmer for 15 minutes, and then stir in the seafood and spinach to heat through. Season to taste.

Lamb with barley

Serves 4

  2 tbsp rapeseed oil
  4 lean lamb shanks
  6 large carrots, peeled and chopped into chunks
  6 shallots, peeled and quartered
  4 cloves garlic, peeled and crushed
  handful of fresh thyme
  1 tbsp tomato purée
  1 tbsp plain flour
  1 litre of chicken stock
  400g/14oz tin can of plum tomatoes
  60g/2 ½oz pearl barley

Preheat the oven to 170°C/340°F/Gas mark 3. Heat the oil in a large casserole and add the lamb. Allow to cook for 10 minutes while it browns all over and then remove and set to one side. Add the carrot, shallots, garlic and thyme and cook for 10 minutes. Then add the tomato purée, flour, stock and tomatoes, stir well and bring to the boil. Simmer for a few minutes and then add the lamb and pearl barley. Cover with a lid and transfer to the oven for 3 hours.

Citrus salmon

Serves 2

  100g/4oz new potatoes, scrubbed
  2 skinless and boneless salmon fillets (approx 150g/5oz each)
  1 tbsp rapeseed oil, plus extra for rubbing

knob of fresh ginger, peeled and grated
½ red chilli, deseeded and finely chopped
2 tsp lemongrass paste
2 spring onions, chopped
juice of 1 lemon
2 large handfuls of fresh coriander/cilantro, chopped
1 bag of mixed salad leaves
1 tbsp sunflower seeds

Bring a large pan of salted water to the boil and add the new potatoes. Return to the boil, reduce the heat and simmer for 15 minutes, or until just cooked through. Set aside to cool.

Rub the salmon fillets with a little oil and place a non-stick frying pan over a high heat. Sear the salmon for 10 minutes, turning regularly until golden and cooked through. Set aside to cool.

Make a dressing by whisking together the oil, ginger, chilli, lemongrass paste, spring onions and lemon juice.

Break up the salmon fillets into bite-sized chunks and lightly crush the new potatoes with the back of a spoon, then toss together and season well. Arrange the fish and potatoes on top of the leaves, scatter on the seeds and drizzle on the dressing.

Shopping list
2 pints of milk/almond milk (or 1 of each)
Large pot of Greek yogurt
1 punnet of berries
2 bananas
12 eggs (7 used this week)
1 grapefruit
2 red onions

5 red peppers

1 pack of chorizo

1 bag of spinach leaves

1 bag of new potatoes

1 small celeriac

1 red chilli

1 avocado

1 lime

3 lemons

1 smoked mackerel fillet

Bunch of spring onions

Bunch each of fresh herbs – chives, parsley, mint, coriander/
cilantro, thyme

1 golden beetroot

1 orange

1 apple

1 chicory

Tomatoes

2 chicken drumsticks

1 pork fillet

1 pack of tenderstem broccoli

1 sweet potato

1 fennel bulb

250g/9oz bag mixed seafood

4 lamb shanks

8 carrots

2 salmon steaks

250g/9oz white fish

Leftover from last week

Feta

Celery

Crème fraiche
Watercress

Store cupboard
Large tin of baby corn
1 tin black-eyed beans
1 jar of horseradish sauce
1 tin of haricot/navy beans
1 tin of water chestnuts
2 tins of tomatoes
Pearl barley
Lemongrass paste
Pistachio nuts
Spices – Cajun spice

WEEK 4

Grilled fruit with nuts and yoghurt

Serves 2
For the marinade:
2 tbsp honey
1 tsp olive oil
1 tbsp fresh lime juice
1 tsp ground cinnamon
1 ripe pineapple, peeled and cut into half inch slices
50g/2oz raspberries
2 tbsp hazelnuts, roughly chopped
handful of mint leaves, torn
Greek yoghurt to serve

In a small bowl, combine the honey, olive oil, lime juice and cinnamon and whisk to blend. Lightly brush the pineapple slices with the marinade. Place under a hot grill, turning once and basting once or twice with the remaining marinade, until tender and golden, about 3–5 minutes on each side.

Serve 2 slices, scattered with the raspberries, hazelnuts and mint and a large dollop of yoghurt.

Muffin stack

Serves 2
  2 wholemeal English muffins, split and toasted
  2 slices (approx 50g) smoked salmon
  1 tbsp crème fraiche
  1 tsp hot horseradish sauce or mustard
  squeeze of lemon juice
  2 radishes, thinly sliced
  2 handfuls of watercress, chopped
  2 eggs, poached
  1 tbsp pine nuts, toasted

Place a slice of smoked salmon on each half of the muffin. Mix together the crème fraiche, horseradish sauce or mustard and lemon juice and spread over the salmon. Top with the slices of radish, a handful of watercress and a poached egg and a scatter of pine nuts.

Prawn pho

Serves 2
  1 litre of vegetable stock
  1 small tin water chestnuts, drained and rinsed
  50g/2oz baby corn
  1 bag of beansprouts
  50g/2oz mangetout/snow peas
  50g/2oz sugar snap peas
  knob of ginger, peeled and grated
  1 tsp honey
  1 tbsp fish sauce
  juice of half a lime
  12 large prawns, shelled and deveined
  handful each of fresh basil leaves, mint, coriander/cilantro
  ½ red chilli, finely sliced

Pour the stock into a large saucepan and bring to the boil, add the chestnuts, sweetcorn, beansprouts, mangetout/snow peas and peas and cook for 3–4 minutes. Add the honey, fish sauce and lime juice, ginger and season. Cook prawns in the broth until pink, about 2–3 minutes. Add herbs and red chilli to serve.

Pea dip

Makes 2–3 portions (will keep in the fridge for 2–3 days)
  100g/4oz frozen petits pois
  100g/4oz frozen soya beans
  100g/4oz artichoke hearts (from a jar), drained
  2 tsp ground cumin

2 tbsp lemon juice
4 tbsp olive oil
small handful of mint leaves
salt and freshly ground black pepper

Tip the peas and soya beans into a bowl and pour over boiling water to cover. Leave for 5 minutes, then drain well and tip into a food processor. Add all the remaining ingredients and pulse to make a rough purée. Season to taste and then spoon into a serving bowl. Cover with cling film and chill until ready to serve.

Chicken and butter bean salad

Serves 1
  1 skinless chicken breast
  50g/2oz asparagus, tough ends snapped off and discarded
  ½ red pepper, deseeded and thinly sliced
  olive oil, for drizzling
  2 tbsp Greek yoghurt
  1 tbsp crème fraiche
  Juice of half a lemon
  ½ clove garlic, crushed
  1 tbsp chopped dill
  2 handfuls of mixed salad leaves
  200g/7oz tinned butter beans/lima beans, drained and rinsed
  1 tbsp pine nuts, toasted
  salt and freshly ground black pepper

Preheat the oven to 220°C/430°F/Gas mark 7. Arrange the chicken, asparagus and red pepper in a large, shallow roasting tin and drizzle with olive oil to coat. Season well and then roast in the oven for 20 minutes, stirring halfway through, until the chicken is cooked through and the vegetables are tender and starting to caramelize. Allow the chicken to cool and when cool enough to handle, roughly shred.

In a small bowl, whisk together the yogurt, crème fraiche, lemon juice, garlic and dill to make a dressing. Season to taste.

Place the leaves in a tub, add the butter beans/lima beans, chicken and veg and scatter over the pine nuts, add the dressing and toss together.

Salsa verde

Makes enough for 2–3 meals
  3 tbsp roughly chopped fresh mint
  3 tbsp torn fresh basil
  3 tbsp roughly chopped flat-leaf parsley
  1 shallot, roughly chopped
  1 clove garlic, roughly chopped
  zest of 1 lemon
  2 tbsp capers, drained
  4 anchovies, roughly chopped
  ½ tsp mustard
  3 tbsp olive oil

Use a pestle and mortar to roughly crush everything together.

Chicken soba noodles

Serves 2
  2 bundles soba noodles (about 200g)
  2 tbsp rapeseed oil

½ red chilli, deseeded and finely sliced
50g /2oz, tenderstem broccoli
1 carrot, cut into matchsticks
50g /2oz, mangetout/snow peas, finely sliced
150g /5oz, shredded cooked chicken
1 tbsp sesame seeds
handful of cashew nuts
splash of soy sauce

Cook the noodles in boiling water, according to the packet instructions. Drain well. Heat the oil in a wok and allow to get very hot before adding the chilli, broccoli, carrot and mangetout/snow peas. Stir fry for a couple of minutes and then add the shredded chicken and noodles, allow to heat through and then when ready to serve, scatter over the sesame seeds and cashew nuts and the soy sauce.

Shopping list
2 pints of milk/almond milk (or 1 of each)
Large pot of Greek yogurt
1 punnet of berries
2 bananas
1 grapefruit
2 limes
1 pineapple
1 punnet of raspberries
2 wholemeal English muffins
1 bag of watercress
1 pack of smoked salmon
1 tub of crème fraiche
2 lemons
12 large prawns

1 red chilli
1 mixed pack of mangetout/snow peas, baby sweetcorn and sugar snap peas
1 bag of bean sprouts
Bunch each of fresh herbs – mint, coriander/cilantro, dill, basil, parsley
2 chicken breasts
Bunch of asparagus
Sardines

Leftover from last week

Eggs
Tenderstem broccoli
Radishes
Ginger
Red pepper
Shallots
Carrots
Cucumber
Garlic

Store cupboard

Pine nuts
1 tin of water chestnuts
1 200g/7oz tin of butter beans/lima beans
1 bag of frozen peas
1 jar of artichoke hearts
1 tin of anchovies
Soba noodles

With your diet plan covered, it's time to turn our attention to exercise. In Chapter Nine, Peta outlines the four-week exercise plans.

THE FOUR-WEEK AGELESS BODY EXERCISE PLANS

Even the word 'exercise' can be off-putting if you've never tried it or have put it on the back-burner for years. Fear not. This routine is neither time-consuming nor boring. What's more, it will create such rapid transformation to your body (and self-esteem) that you will wonder why you ever put off doing it in the first place.

WHERE TO START

There are three phases to the exercise plan – groundwork (the beginner phase), progression (phase 2) and maintenance (phase 3). It is advisable to work your way through all three levels, although if you have already been doing plenty of interval training you might wish to skip 'groundwork' and head straight to 'progression'. If, at the end of each phase, you feel that the workload is still too challenging, then by all means re-do that particular phase. You're cheating nobody but yourself by rushing through them. Gradual progression is important; there's no race to achieve an ageless body. Indeed, doing too much too soon can backfire.

How often?

Each phase is based on four workout days a week. They needn't be done on the days prescribed although it is best to stick loosely to the format and preferably not to do all of your workouts, binge-fashion, on consecutive days. Although the remaining weekdays are designated 'rest' days, this doesn't mean you should sit in the parked position doing nothing. As we've seen, integrating activity into your daily life is really important in your quest for an ageless body, so pack in as much walking, standing, stair-climbing as possible whenever you can. You may find that you like the routine of a scheduled workout and that you miss it on the days it's not timetabled. If that's the case, there is the option of adding in the following 'rest day' activities when you feel like it. They are by no means obligatory:

Beginner: 20 minutes gentle cardio or 15 minutes stretching.

Intermediate: 20–30 minutes moderate cardio or 20 minutes stretching.

Advanced: 30–40 minutes moderate cardio or 20 minutes stretching.

How long?

The really good news is that none of the scheduled sessions last longer than 45 minutes. At 'groundwork' level, you can expect to be working out for no more than 20 minutes at a time. What matters as we age is intensity and, of course, consistency.

WHAT DOES IT ENTAIL?

As you have read, achieving an Ageless Body does not require you to hammer away on gym equipment every day, nor does it mean lengthy aerobic slogs. In fact, both approaches can be counter-productive. What is needed at this stage of life is a refined and focused plan that will fit neatly into your lifestyle and not leave you too knackered to juggle everything else.

That doesn't mean effort required is minimal. Far from it. You'll be working hard, but for shorter periods of time than many of you will be used to. And progression will be gentle so that you should be ready to move onwards and upwards in accordance with the schedules.

In the 'groundwork' phase, you will be introduced to elements of interval training that will boost your cardiovascular fitness and get you used to pushing yourself to new limits in short bursts. Some strength and conditioning exercises will also be added to the end of that phase.

In the 'progression' phase, things will be ramped up. Now that you have a good base level of fitness, more strength work with weights, calisthenics (body weight exercises) and mini-circuits will be introduced in addition to the interval training you started in the first phase.

By the time you embark on the 'maintenance' phase, your body will have changed beyond recognition. You'll feel and look younger – which, of course is our goal – so the emphasis switches to keeping things on that even keel. Some variety will be added so that you don't get bored and by the time you complete the plan you will be armed with enough fitness knowledge to keep holding back the years yourself.

All of the exercises are described in Chapter Ten.

CARDIO INTENSITY

Gentle: A manageable pace at which you can easily hold a conversation.

Steady: Feels like you are making more effort, but you can still chat.

Moderate: Pick up the pace to a level where you can chat only sporadically.

Hard: No chatting at this level. It's all-out effort.

LINGO

Fitness language is a law unto itself, constantly evolving and always prone to catching you out with the latest terminology. Our exercise plans feature five main sessions: Cardio; Long HIIT; Short HIIT; Calisthenics; and Weight Blasters. Here's a brief explanation of the terms along with a couple of other phrases it is useful to know. Beyond these, there is little you need to remember.

Cardio (or cardiovascular activity): This is the kind that works your heart and lungs, and is integral to all levels of the programme. There are numerous choices here – the key is to pick one you enjoy. No other rules apply. Believe me, forcing yourself to slog away on a rowing machine or cross trainer when it's an activity you loathe is no fun at all. Mix and match is the best approach as it provides variety for both muscles and mind.

Reps (or repetitions): The number of exercises you need to do in a 'set' (see below).

Sets: The number of 'groups' of exercises that comprise a workout.

Long HIIT: High Intensity Interval Training. We've called it Long HIIT because it entails cardio activity and comprises a session lasting anything from 12–30 minutes. Not *that* long.

Short HIIT: Similar to above, only an even shorter, faster burst of effort using more strength-based exercises followed by a timed recovery.

Abs: Abdominal muscles. Exercises to work these are included throughout the plan.

Calisthenics: Exercises using only your own body weight for resistance.

Weight Blasters: Exercises using resistance and weights to build strength and tone.

EQUIPMENT

The good news is you don't need to spend a small fortune on exercise equipment, neither do you need to join a gym. For the most part, the Ageless Body workout plans require few accessories, but you will need to purchase some of the following:

Set of dumbbells: Even the word 'weights' scares many people. But if you are still dubious about the benefits that resistance and strength training have for your body, please re-read Part One of the book. Weights are essential for the workout plans that follow. So, what to buy? There are two basic categories of dumbbell: those that have weights you can add or remove to a single bar, and sets of dumbbells of different weights. For a variety of reasons, I recommend the former. Weights sets take up a lot of space and are generally more expensive. How heavy your weights should be is dependent on your experience and strength as well as your build. Most people start with a 3–4kg weighted dumbbell, progressing to 6kg and 9kg as they get fitter and stronger. It's important your weights aren't too light – you should be able to manage no more than the number of repetitions prescribed in each workout, otherwise your weight is too light. If you are struggling to complete the reps, you will need to reduce the load for a while.

Stopwatch: Sports watches and fitness trackers come with all sorts of functions these days. I've tried more than many and can honestly say the only setting I routinely use is the stopwatch or timer. GPS functions are useful, but unreliable in that they require a signal before they whirr into action. To cut to the chase, I'd save your money and invest in a plain, bog-standard stopwatch without any of the high tech trimmings.

Trainers: It's worth bearing in mind these have a shelf life and the pair that's been lurking in the back of your wardrobe for several years are probably past their sell-by date. If running is a cardio activity of choice, then you'll need a decent and supportive pair of specialist trainers (visit a running shop for these if you are unsure what to buy). Otherwise cross trainers or a regular pair of training shoes will suffice. Brands I love include Asics, Brooks, Hoka One and New Balance. Don't buy into the barefoot 'footglove' trend unless you have been wearing them for a while. Physios have reported a sharp hike in injuries among people who ditch regular shoes with cushioning for these, unaware that their legs and feet lack the muscle strength needed to support the body when wearing them.

Waterproof clothing: Another must-buy if you plan to do any outdoor activity. From experience I can confirm that no investment is as worthwhile as a good, breathable waterproof jacket and, if you are a runner or walker, waterproof shoes. Gore-Tex fabrics are ideal for outwear although most of the large sports manufacturers produce their own version. As for shoes, trail running shoes are your best bet (they do tend to be a little less flexible and take a bit of getting used to at first) and my most trusty pair is from Salomon. When wearing them I have yet to return from a run, however wet the ground, with soggy socks.

Sports bra: Essential if you want to avoid further boob-droop. It never ceases to amaze me how few women invest in a decent sports bra. All that jiggling beneath a tee-shirt is asking for the breast tissue to be stretched beyond what is reasonable. As any woman bigger than a B-cup will tell you, the trauma of taming an unwieldy cleavage in order to complete a workout is worthy of high tech investigation.

With no muscle and only the fragile outer skin and connective tissues called Cooper's Ligaments providing support, breasts are a law unto themselves when it comes to movement, swaying and bobbing independently of the torso. A series of experiments by the University of Portsmouth's Breast Health research group headed by Dr Joanna Scurr have charted the trajectory of women's breasts using infrared cameras and found that they don't merely bounce up and down, but move through a complicated figure of eight pattern when a woman runs or walks [64].

Unconstrained, each breast swung as much as 8 inches (21cm) in space during activity on a treadmill and even when wearing a standard sports bra, Dr Scurr and her team showed there was still considerable oscillation. The more vigorous the workout, the more mobile the appendages become – so running causes more sway than walking. And since the average breast weighs 7–10oz (10.6g), the level of discomfort and the potential for embarrassment rise accordingly. Reducing speed from a sprint to a jog has little effect on lessening bounce. Too much bouncing eventually causes irreversible sag as the delicate structure is strained to its limits, more so as you get older.

Unsurprisingly, manufacturers are revelling in the emergence of such findings and the discovery that breasts carry such weight in the world of science. The market for the once humble and slightly greying sports bra is booming.

Being generously busted myself, I've spent years researching what's on offer. What I've discovered is that sports bras come in various incarnations, but most fall into one of two categories: compression – the kind that bandage boobs to flatten them against the chest; and encapsulation, that cradle each breast individually. My all-time favourite is the Shock Absorber Ultimate Run range that really does seem to hold everything in place. When it was rigorously tested at the University of Portsmouth, the bra was found to reduce bounce in joggers by 78 per cent compared with ordinary bras.

If you are very large busted, the Lynx sports bra is worth a try. Designed by Cynthia Smith, an American molecular scientist and marathon runner, it is unique in its patented construction that supports from the sides instead of the usual shoulder straps and band. In pilot studies involving women size DD-to G-cup at Loughborough University, its 'bounce factor' outperformed rival bras by providing a more comfortable workout. Other good brands include Anita and Panache. All are available from the fabulously named lessbounce.com or boobydoo.co.uk.

Gym ball: These are excellent for resistance work with one caveat – where to keep them once they've been inflated. So, although there are exercises in the programme that use them, they are not obligatory and alternatives are given. If you do choose to buy one, opt for a 25-inch (65 cm) ball, which can be bought for very little from shops like Argos.

THE PLANS

1

DAY ONE

Groundwork: 15 minutes steady cardio followed by 4 x 10 second sprints

Progression: Short HIIT: that's 20 seconds of an exercise from the HIIT list (see pp. 220–4) followed by 40 seconds rest, repeated for 5 minutes

Maintenance: Calisthenic Circuit: select three exercises from the list on pp. 232–7 (choosing some upper and some lower body moves) and perform 10 repetitions of each in succession (no rest).
Take a 40 second break and repeat four times in total.

2

DAY TWO

Groundwork: Active rest

Progression: 5 minutes gentle cardio, then the following Calisthenics Circuit:
    Alternate lunges x 15 each leg
    Single leg body lifts x 12 each leg
    Step-ups x 15 each leg
    Hamstring curls x 15
    Push-ups x 15 (or to failure)
Repeat the exercises twice with 50 seconds rest between each set.
    Plank x 40 seconds (or to failure)

Maintenance: 30 minutes steady cardio (optional)

DAY THREE

Groundwork: 5 minutes gentle cardio; 5 x (1 minute hard cardio, followed by 1 minute gentle cardio); 5 minutes gentle cardio

Progression: Active rest

Maintenance: Active rest

4

DAY FOUR

Groundwork: Active rest

Progression: 20 minutes steady cardio followed by:
  Ab crunches x 30
  Knee crossovers x 15 each leg
  V-sits x 20
  Plank x 30 seconds, or to failure

Maintenance: Weight Burner Circuit:
  Lateral raise x 12
  Weighted lunges x 12 each leg
  Shoulder press x 12
  Triceps kick back x 12 each arm
  Weighted calf raise x 15
  Weighted side bend x 12 each side
*Repeat the circuit three times with 40 seconds recovery
between each set.*

DAY FIVE

Groundwork: 5 minutes gentle cardio, 10 minutes moderate cardio, 5 minutes gentle cardio

Progression: Active rest

Maintenance: 25 minutes steady cardio followed by Ab Circuit:
 Gym ball plank x 40 seconds
 Superman x 30 seconds
 V-sits x 25
 Wood chopper x 12 each side

6

DAY SIX

Groundwork: Active rest

Progression: 5 minutes gentle cardio followed by Weight Burner Circuit:
   Triceps dips x 15 (or to failure)
   Upright row x 12
   Pullovers x 12
   Shoulder press x 12
   Single arm fly x 12 each side
   Bicep curl x 12 each arm
Repeat the above routine twice with a 40 second rest between sets.

Maintenance: Active rest

7

DAY SEVEN

Groundwork: Long HIIT: 16 minutes steady cardio followed by 4 x 10 second sprints

Progression: Active rest

Maintenance: 8 minutes of HIIT; that's 20 seconds of an exercise from the HIIT list (see pp. 220–4) followed by 40 seconds rest, repeated for 8 minutes

8

DAY EIGHT

Groundwork: Long HIIT: 6 minutes steady cardio;
6 x (30 seconds hard cardio, 30 seconds gentle cardio);
6 minutes gentle cardio

Progression: Short HIIT: that's 20 seconds of an exercise
from the HIIT list (see pp. 220–4), followed by 40
seconds rest, repeated for a total of 5 minutes

Maintenance: Active rest

DAY NINE

Groundwork: Active rest

Progression: Active rest

Maintenance: Calisthenics Circuit: select three exercises from the list (choosing some upper and some lower body moves, see pp. 232–7) and perform 10 repetitions of each in succession (no rest).
Take a 40 second break and repeat four times in total.

10

DAY TEN

Groundwork: 18 minutes steady cardio followed by 4 x 10 second sprints

Progression: 5 minutes gentle cardio, then the following Calisthenics Circuit:
    Sumo squats x 15
    Lateral lunges x 12
    Single leg bridge x 15 seconds each leg
    Push-ups x 16 (or to failure)
    Oblique crunches x 30
Repeat the exercises twice with a 50 second rest between sets.

Maintenance: 10 minutes moderate cardio, 5 minutes steady, 10 minutes moderate, 5 minutes steady, followed by Ab Circuit:
    Oblique plank x 40 seconds each side
    Oblique crunches x 30 each side
    Knee crossover tucks x 15 each side
    Russian Twist x 12 each side

DAY ELEVEN

Groundwork: Active rest

Progression: Active rest

Maintenance: Active rest

12

DAY TWELVE

Groundwork: Long HIIT: 6 minutes steady cardio;
6 x (40 seconds hard cardio, 20 seconds gentle cardio);
6 minutes gentle cardio

Progression: 20 minutes steady cardio followed by
Ab Circuit:
  Oblique crunches x 30
  Oblique plank x 30 seconds each side (or to failure)
  Woodchopper x 15 each side
  Russian Twist x 20

Maintenance: Weight Burner Circuit:
  Single arm fly x 12 each arm
  Arnold press x 12
  Gym ball plank x 40 seconds
  Upright row x 15
  Pullovers x 15
  Weighted lunges x 15 each leg
Repeat circuit three times with 40 seconds rest between
set each.

13

DAY THIRTEEN

Groundwork: Active rest

Progression: 5 minutes gentle cardio, followed by
Weight Burner Circuit:
  Lateral raise x 15
  Arnold press x 15
  Reverse fly x 12
  Pullovers x 12
  Bicep curl x 12 each arm
  Upright row x 15
Repeat the routine twice with 40 seconds rest between
each set.

Maintenance: 35 minutes steady cardio (optional)

14

DAY FOURTEEN

Groundwork: 20 minutes moderate cardio, followed by 4 x 10 second sprints

Progression: Active rest

Maintenance: 8 minutes of Short HIIT; that's 20 seconds of an exercise from the HIIT list (see pp. 220–4) followed by 40 seconds rest, repeated for 8 minutes

15

DAY FIFTEEN

Groundwork: 5 minutes gentle cardio, 10 minutes steady cardio, 5 minutes gentle cardio, followed by 30 x ab crunches, 30 seconds plank, 20 x V-sits, 30 x oblique crunches

Progression: 5 minutes gentle cardio, then the following Long HIIT; 40 seconds hard, 20 seconds gentle cardio for 7 minutes; 5 minutes gentle cardio

Maintenance: Active rest

16

DAY SIXTEEN

Groundwork: Active rest

Progression: 5 minutes gentle cardio, then the following Calisthenics Circuit:
    Alternate lunges x 15 each leg
    Push-ups x 16, or to failure
    Squats x 15
    Hamstring curls x 15
    Step-ups x 15 each leg
    Plank x 40 seconds, or to failure
Repeat the circuit three times with a 50 second rest between each set.

Maintenance: Calisthenics Circuit: select three exercises from the list (choosing some upper and some lower body moves, see pp. 232–7) and perform 10 repetitions of each in succession (no rest).
Take a 40 second break and repeat four times in total.

DAY SEVENTEEN

Groundwork: 5 minutes gentle cardio, then Long HIIT: 5 x (1 minute hard cardio, 1 minute gentle cardio); 5 minutes steady cardio; 20 x squats; 20 x walking lunges; 20 x step-ups each leg

Progression: Active rest

Maintenance: 10 minutes moderate cardio, 15 minutes steady cardio, 10 minutes moderate followed by Ab Circuit:
Ab crunches x 30
Plank x 40 seconds
V-sits x 20
Single leg bridge x 15 seconds each side

18

DAY EIGHTEEN

Groundwork: Active rest

Progression: 20 minutes steady cardio followed by
Ab Circuit:
    Plank x 40 seconds, or to failure
    Ab crunch x 30
    Oblique ab crunch x 15 each side
    V-sits x 20

Maintenance: Active rest

19

DAY NINETEEN

Groundwork: 5 minutes gentle cardio, 10 minutes moderate cardio, 5 minutes steady cardio followed by: 12 x push-ups; 15 x triceps dips; 15 x upright row

Progression: 5 minutes gentle cardio followed by Weight Burner Circuit:
   Triceps dips x 15 (or to failure)
   Upright row x 12
   Pullovers x 12
   Shoulder press x 12
   Single arm fly x 12 each side
   Bicep curl x 12 each arm
Repeat the above routine three times with a 40 second rest between sets.

Maintenance: Weight Burner Circuit:
   Triceps kick back x 12
   Weighted calf raise x 15
   Bent over row x 12 each arm
   Weighted side bend x 12 each side
   Single arm fly x 12 each arm
   Shoulder press x 12
Repeat each circuit three times with a 40 second rest between sets.

20

DAY TWENTY

Groundwork: Active rest

Progression: Active rest

Maintenance: 40 minutes steady cardio (optional)

21

DAY TWENTY-ONE

Groundwork: 5 minutes steady cardio followed by Long HIIT: 6 x (30 seconds hard cardio, 30 seconds gentle cardio), 5 minutes gentle cardio; 20 x knee tucks, 20 seconds oblique plank (each side), 20 x oblique crunches, 10 seconds x single leg body lift (each side)

Progression: Active rest

Maintenance: 8 minutes of HIIT; that's 20 seconds of an exercise from the HIIT list (see pp. 220–4) followed by 40 seconds rest repeated for 8 minutes

22

DAY TWENTY-TWO

Groundwork: Active rest

Progression: Calisthenics Circuit:
   Single leg body lift x 12 each leg
   Sumo squats x 15
   Lateral lunges x 12 each leg
   Wall squats x 40 seconds (or to failure)
   Oblique plank x 30 seconds (or to failure)
   Step-ups x 15 seconds each leg
*Repeat the circuit three times with a 50 second rest between
each set.*

Maintenance: Active rest

23

DAY TWENTY-THREE

Groundwork: 6 minutes gentle cardio followed by Long HIIT: 6 x (60 seconds hard cardio, 60 seconds gentle), 6 minutes steady cardio; 20 seconds x wall squats, 20 x walking lunges, 20 x step-ups (each leg)

Progression: 20 minutes moderate cardio or active rest

Maintenance: Calisthenics Circuit: select four exercises from the list (choosing some upper and some lower body moves, see pp. 232–7) and perform 10 repetitions of each in succession (no rest).
Take a 40 second break and repeat four times in total.

24

DAY TWENTY-FOUR

Groundwork: Active rest

Progression: Active rest

Maintenance: 10 minutes moderate cardio, 5 minutes steady, 10 minutes moderate, 5 minutes steady, followed by Ab Circuit:
    Oblique plank x 40 seconds each side
    Oblique crunches x 30 each side
    Knee crossover tucks x 15 each side
    Russian Twist x 12 each side

25

DAY TWENTY-FIVE

Groundwork: 5 minutes gentle cardio, 5 minutes steady cardio, 5 minutes hard cardio, 5 minutes gentle cardio; 12 x push-ups; 15 x triceps overhead extension; 15 x shoulder press

Progression: 25 minutes steady cardio followed by Ab Circuit:
  Russian Twist x 20
  Oblique plank x 40 seconds each side (or to failure)
  Single leg bridge x 15 each side
  Knee crossovers x 15 each side

Maintenance: Active rest

26

DAY TWENTY-SIX

Groundwork: Active rest

Progression: Active rest

Maintenance: Weight Burner circuit:
  Lateral raise x 12
  Weighted lunges x 12 each leg
  Shoulder press x 12
  Triceps kick back x 12 each arm
  Weighted calf raise x 15
  Weighted side bend x 12 each side
Repeat the circuit three times with 40 seconds recovery between each set.

DAY TWENTY-SEVEN

Groundwork: 30 x ab crunches, 30 seconds oblique plank (each side), 20 x V-sits, 30 x oblique crunches

Progression: 5 minutes gentle cardio followed by:
    Lateral raise x 15
    Arnold press x 15
    Reverse fly x 12
    Pullovers x 12
    Bicep curl x 12 each arm
    Upright row x 15
Repeat the routine three times with 40 seconds rest between each set.

Maintenance: 45 minutes steady cardio (optional) or rest.

28

DAY TWENTY-EIGHT

Groundwork: Active rest

Progression: 5 minutes of HIIT with mountain climbers: 20 seconds of mountain climbers, 40 seconds rest, repeated for 5 minutes

Maintenance: 8 minutes of HIIT; that's 20 seconds of an exercise from the HIIT list (see pp. 220–4), followed by 40 seconds rest repeated for 8 minutes

DAY TWENTY-NINE

Groundwork: 4 minutes gentle cardio, 4 minutes hard cardio, 4 minutes gentle cardio; 2 minutes hard cardio, 4 minutes gentle cardio; 20 x sumo squats, 20 x walking lunges, 20 x step-ups (each leg)

Progression: Active rest

Maintenance: Active rest

30

DAY THIRTY

Groundwork: 20 minutes moderate cardio; 4 x 10 second sprints

Progression: 5 minutes gentle cardio; 30 seconds hard cardio, 30 seconds gentle cardio for 7 minutes; 5 minutes gentle cardio

Maintenance: Calisthenics Circuit: select four exercises from the list (choosing some upper and some lower body moves see pp. 232–7) and perform 10 repetitions of each in succession (no rest).
Take a 40 second break and repeat four times in total.

Now all you need to know is how to do the exercises. That will be covered in the chapter that follows.

CHAPTER TEN

THE EXERCISES

To keep things simple (who wants a workout programme so complex that you struggle to understand it, let alone follow it?), we have grouped all of the exercises you will do in the Ageless Body workouts into six basic types: Cardio, Long HIIT, Short HIIT, Weight Burners, Calisthenics and Abs. By the end of the three-month programme you will hopefully have become so familiar with what each entails that you will probably not need to refer to the book much at all. At least, that's our aim. We hope the Ageless Body plan will become second nature, something you do instinctively because you know it works. In the meantime, here's an overview of each exercise, how it will help you reach your goals and a 'how to' for each of the exercises you'll be trying:

CARDIO
The basics

As research has emerged showing that short, sharp sessions are highly effective at fat-burning, toning and general fitness-boosting, so cardiovascular (cardio) workouts have fallen out of favour in the gym world. Whereas the 1980s and 1990s were all about how long you spent exercising, now the focus is on how little time you can get away with. However, there's a balance to achieve, and with science showing that endurance activity boosts cardio health and the enhanced functioning of our heart and lungs, our belief is that it is essential for all-round results.

Our workout plan includes cardio sessions lasting up to 45 minutes. There is no rule stating you can't do more occasionally. I love nothing more than a long run when I need some time to myself. What isn't necessary in the quest for an Ageless Body is the relentless pursuit of extreme cardio goals. By all means run a marathon or complete a triathlon, but if you are aiming to preserve health, looks and sanity, then do so sparingly.

We've kept the cardio options open. We've made some suggestions, but really the world of endurance activity is your oyster. If skipping or inline skating are more your thing, by all means include them. A word too on cardio gym equipment: most of the cardio machines at the gym can be used for these workouts. Perhaps the most efficient (treadmills, rowing machines and bikes aside) is the cross trainer, but if you are a gym bunny, feel free to mix and match to suit your needs.

Walking: We tend to look down on walking, to deride it as a poor relation to running because of its lesser ability to burn calories and emit a sweat. Yet it really has come into its own as an essential element of the older A-lister's exercise regimen. Charlize Theron, Uma Thurman and Eva Mendes are among those who credit walking with helping them to stay in shape.

It's hard to find an Ageless Body activity with a greater celebrity following or, indeed, the barrage of research that walking has to support it. It's been shown to reduce cancer death risk by up to 34 per cent and cut your risk of Type 2 diabetes in half. Regular brisk walking can lower your risk of high blood pressure, high cholesterol and diabetes as much as running can, according to a six-year study published in the American Heart Association's journal *Arteriosclerosis, Thrombosis and Vascular Biology* [65]. It is also weight bearing so helps strengthen bones that begin to lose mass as we age, lowering the risk of osteoporosis. And, of course, it's great for those with vulnerable joints. Studies at the University of Wisconsin have shown that, compared with running, even a vigorous walk reduces impact on vulnerable hips, ankles and knees by 26 per cent [66].

And the improvements come thick and fast with the more walking you do. Researchers reporting in *The Lancet* medical journal found that adding 2000 moderately paced walking steps (or 20 minutes) a day to regular activity could help people to cut their risk of heart attacks and strokes by 8 per cent. Doing 4000 more steps (40 minutes of added walking) matches the gains obtained from taking cholesterol-lowering drugs [67].

Three weekly walks of 45 minutes have been shown to reduce symptoms of Parkinson's disease and a study funded by Kidney Research UK and conducted at the University of Leicester found that walking for half an hour on three to five days a week, significantly reduced kidney disease symptoms, including tiredness and joint pain, in a group of patients preparing to undergo dialysis [68]. It's what it does for your mind, though, that swings it for many. Walk outside, as most of us do, and you don't just get a crucial dose of health-boosting vitamin D, but the mental gains are colossal. Scottish researchers found that outdoor exercise, including a stroll, had a 50 per cent greater positive effect on mental health than going to the gym and it's also been associated with plummeting levels of tension, anger and depression.

The draw for us, though, is that you can walk without gadgets and fancy footwork. Both Sarah and I walk everywhere – to meetings, school, the park. A comfortable pair of trainers or shoes along with a well-fitted backpack if you plan a more serious jaunt is all that's needed to get going. It requires no gym membership and it can become part of your routine wherever you live – researchers have shown that city dwellers tend to walk 15 minutes a day more than suburbanites because they leave their cars at home. It requires no instruction – we can all do it – and, of course, it gives you a huge fat-burning advantage.

Running: For every reason you hear not to run in middle age and beyond, there is one to prove that you should. Running is a number one favourite activity of both Sarah and myself. We couldn't live without it. And, in fact, we are encouraged that we could live longer by doing it. Despite the scare stories that the activity is a shortcut to heart disease and unreliable joints, researchers have shown that it can extend our lives rather than cut them short.

A landmark study by the University of California compared the long-term health of a group of running club members aged 50-plus with another group of healthy non-runners, believing the fitness habit might leave the joggers crippled with health problems. On the contrary, after 20 years, 34 per cent of the non-runners had died compared with 15 per cent of the runners, and the surviving joggers were generally in better health overall [69].

Findings presented by the American College of Sports Medicine suggested that regular running lowered the risk of dying early so long as no more than 20 miles (32km) in up to five sessions a week were covered, in trainers and at a speed no faster than 5–7 miles (8–11km) per hour. Of around 53,000 adults in that study, those who ran further and faster or more often were no worse off than non-runners when it came to longevity but 'seemed to lose the survival advantage gained at lower doses of running' [70].

When it comes to the knees, rumours abound of how running can wreck them. For the most part these rumours are exaggerated and inaccurate. Usually, it's not running in itself that causes problems, but bad habits and erratic running habits along with underlying injuries from other sports. A 2013 study of almost 75,000 adult runners reported finding 'no evidence that running increases the risk of osteoarthritis, including participation in marathons' [71]. In fact, those who ran regularly were at less risk of developing knee arthritis than less active counterparts. It backed up findings from a previous 21-year study at Stamford University which tracked nearly 1000 running club members and non-runners and found no difference in the state of their knees at the end of the investigation [72].

One thing we've noticed among middle-aged runners is a fixation with technique. We would all like to have the seemingly effortless running style of someone like Seb Coe in his prime. Unfortunately, most of us are not made to run that way. The good news is that it doesn't matter as much as you've probably been led to believe.

The best advice is to find the running style that suits your body. Correcting obvious howlers such as a nodding head (puts strain on the back), hunched shoulders (inhibits stride length) and swinging arms or flicking-out feet (puts strain on the hips and knees) is helpful, but the stronger and fitter you get, the more you will find your running style corrects itself. Indeed, researchers at the University of Exeter's human performance group showed that we actually self-adjust our style just by running more [73]. They studied a group of women who had recently taken up running and after several weeks found they were naturally bending their knees and flexing their ankles slightly more – good news for injury avoidance.

Cycling: By far the fastest growing group on two wheels, is the middle-aged who are switching to the sport in their droves. There are now about three times as many regular cyclists as there are regular golfers, says Sport England, a massive change from just 20 years ago. Part of the reason is it is kind on joints that have previously been hammered by other activities.

But it is certainly up there with the big players when it comes to boosting fitness. The quadriceps, hamstring, calf and gluteal muscles in the legs and buttocks perform the bulk of the cyclist's work – which is good news because these large muscle groups burn more calories than smaller muscles like the biceps. Even coasting along you can expect to burn 90 calories in 30 minutes. Add some hills or bursts of speed to turn your bike ride into a real workout and you are looking at 200 calories in 30 minutes.

As for boosting your long-term health, there are studies to prove the benefits. Dutch researchers questioned more than 30,000 people for a paper published in the *Journal of the American Medical Association*. They discovered that people who did not cycle to work were 39 per cent more likely to die during the 15-year trial [74]. Meanwhile, researchers at King's College London and the University of Birmingham also revealed how regular cycling can ward off the effects of ageing. Their study of men and women aged 55–79, all of whom cycled regularly, revealed that on almost all measures of physical functioning and fitness, the cyclists didn't show their age [75].

Swimming: As an activity that is kind to our joints and beneficial to our lungs and muscles, swimming is unrivalled. Physiotherapists generally rate it as the best exercise for those with vulnerable joints and injury problems, the water acting as a giant cushion and being much kinder to the joints and tendons than terra firma because it supports your body weight. It's also cheap and easily accessible. Yet far too many of us plod endless lengths of a swimming pool rarely, if ever, changing pace or stroke. The result is a fitness plateau in which this hugely effective cardio exercise never achieves its full potential. It's worthwhile seeking out a stroke improver's course at your local pool if you are less than happy with your technique. It certainly revolutionized my own front crawl, meaning I achieved far greater distances in less time and, frankly, with less effort than I had previously expended puffing and panting my way down every length.

Rowing: Given that it's seen its most dramatic swell in participation among women aged 45-plus in recent years – numbers soaring by almost 40 per cent – it may well be that you have tried this route to a pert bod. Many are spurred on by the fact that the sport is second to none in improving cardiovascular fitness, will tone the legs, upper body and core muscles in one workout and that it burns calories like a furnace. Outdoor rowing is more popular than ever with beginner schemes run by British Rowing.

But even the indoor rower, having long been considered a demon machine, is now usurping the stationary bike as the cardio gym equipment of choice. A growing number of gyms are re-focusing attention on this neglected item of equipment in the form of group rowing classes that are set to take on Spinning in terms of popularity. In New York and LA, indoor rowing classes are a big fitness craze, with gyms having to create waiting lists for group sessions such as Indo-Row and Shock Wave. These sessions are cropping up in gyms here now, and are well worth trying.

Rowing really is in a class of its own when it comes to all-over body-sculpting effects, every stroke requiring you to work the muscles in your calves, upper legs, buttocks, core, upper back and arms. A 50-minute rowing session can gobble 600 calories, more than Spinning because your arms and upper body are used as well. There are other benefits. Rowing is low impact, so easier on delicate knees, hips and ankles than running or military-style circuits.

Good technique is crucial and it really is worth getting someone to talk you through it. It's a common misnomer that the pulling motion makes it an arm-focused workout. In fact, it is particularly good at toning and strengthening the legs and core. Start each stroke by pushing with the legs, not hunching over (power is reduced with a rounded back) and keeping your wrists in line with the handle so that the pulley wire is parallel to the floor.

LONG HIIT

The basics

What we've called Long HIIT is a form of interval training based on the cardio exercises outlined above. There are no rules about which exercise you choose – it's up to you. Variety is best for the mind (and body), but if you loathe cycling, you are simply going to enter a tunnel of misery by embarking on a routine that involves pedalling three times a week, so avoid it.

From the off, in the groundwork phase of the Ageless Body programme you will be incorporating the Long HIIT approach into your weekly exercise and you will soon begin to realize how and why we've made it a cornerstone of the plan. It's not easy, and if it has been some time since you put in a huff and puff level of effort to your workouts, it will take a bit of getting used to, but benefits are reaped extraordinarily quickly.

You'll wonder why you ever thought you needed to spend hours on the treadmill or in the aerobics studio when you can get double the fitness outcome for half or even one-quarter of the input in terms of time. Dozens of studies confirm the benefits of Long (and Short) HIIT. It's particularly good at burning middle-aged fat. Studies looking specifically at groups of volunteers in their forties and fifties have compared long, slow endurance slogs lasting an hour or more with short, intense HIIT sessions and found, time and again, that the abbreviated approach comes up trumps.

In one of several trials at McMaster University in Ontario, subjects were asked to do a session of four to six 30-second bursts with a 4 minute recovery, while a control group plodded away for an hour on the treadmill. This was repeated three times a week for six weeks. At the end of the trial, the joggers had indeed shed some body fat, but the HIIT group had lost double the amount and an impressive 12.4 per cent of their body fat [76].

If it's tough, you might think it makes you ravenously hungry. Not so. In fact, it seems to suppress appetite, at least in the short term, resulting in fewer calories consumed after a workout. A study published in the *International Journal of Obesity* proved this is the case by allowing volunteers to eat as much as they liked after HIIT workouts, moderate exercise or rest [77]. Fewest calories were consumed after the high (621 calories) and very high (594 calories) intensity workouts, compared to the times when they rested (764 extra calories) or did moderate exercise (710 calories).

It works for me. After a long run I might devour a carbohydrate feast; after a Long HIIT session my hunger is curbed for several hours and, even then, I seem to eat more healthily.

SHORT HIIT

The basics

What we refer to as Short HIIT are the sessions that involve a degree of gut-busting effort, but for manageably short bursts. Unless you have been avoiding the gym scene, you might be familiar with the concept of this kind of approach as it has become *the* workout trend of the last few years.

It suits the ageing body for several reasons. Firstly, it is short so your muscles and joints aren't undergoing the kind of intensive hammering that can be detrimental. Secondly, it builds strength and cardiovascular fitness in one conveniently short shot. It is, if you like, an abbreviated form of circuit training that can be done at home with no (or at least very little) equipment.

It's tough and exhausting. But at least it comes in micro-doses. And it produces dramatic results. Let's consider some of the science. Since every pound of muscle uses about 6 calories a day just to sustain itself (and fat a mere 2), it makes sense that your body will become a more efficient user of excess energy if the exercise equation is right. Short HIIT quickly raises metabolic rate, often to levels that can be 15 to 20 times higher than at rest. And, scientists say, this boost continues after you've stopped – the time taken to return to resting levels tends to be dependent on how long and hard you worked.

Exercise scientists at the University of Abertay, Dundee, reported that middle-aged participants who were asked to sprint all out for 6 seconds on a bike then rest for 1 minute, repeating the cycle 10 times, three times a week, improved their fitness levels by as much as 10 per cent in two weeks [78].

Dr John Babraj, who leads the Abertay research group, has conducted other studies on our age group with similarly impressive results – and not just in terms of appearance. His results have shown that, on average, former couch potatoes doing just two 60-second sprints a week lost 2.2lb (1kg) of fat over the two-month trial even though the subjects were asked not to change their usual diet or activity habits. Measures of blood sugar control showed improvements almost matching those of younger people doing more of the same exercise, and the middle-aged subjects also had significantly better cardiovascular function, an important marker of heart disease, after eight weeks [79].

Meanwhile, at Auburn University Montgomery Kinesiology Laboratory in the US, study participants performed a 4-minute Short HIIT session of squat jumps. On average, they blasted away 13.5 calories per minute and doubled their metabolic rates for at least 30 minutes afterward [80]. It would take five times the amount of regular cardio exercise to shed the same number of calories you can in a Short HIIT session, the researchers suggested. Really, what's to lose (other than several pounds of blubber)?

It's worth mentioning the scare stories here as there are plenty of them. As we stated from the outset, it is wise to give yourself an overhaul before starting any new form of exercise. Get things checked out, make sure there are no hidden vulnerabilities creeping up on you with age. With that done, off you go.

Stair climbing: Stairs are widely used by athletes in training, but often overlooked by the rest of us. If you have a decent flight (indoor or out) you can use, then do – they are more effective than the mechanical step-climber and one of the best activities you can do to add tone to your sagging bottom. It's not an easy option. According to the American Lung Foundation, stair running provides the same physical benefits as a run along pavements or flat ground but in half the time. It's perfect for Short HIIT because the descent (walk rather than run down) is ready-made for recovery. Technique matters. Keep your head straight, back upright and use your arms to power you up the steps. Land on the balls of your feet, but make sure you don't hit the edge of the step as

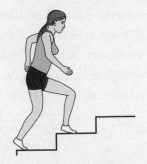

you might wobble and twist an ankle. Unless you are exceptionally long-legged, take every step rather than bounding up two at a time.

Burpees: This one's hard work but will strengthen the whole body. Maintain good technique throughout. Begin by crouching down,

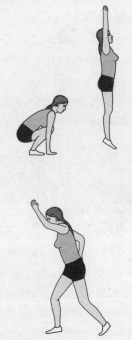

knees tucked into the chest and hands on the floor. Kick back with your feet so that your body forms a press-up position with legs straight and arms straight, in line with the shoulders. Leap into a standing position, getting good height with the jump. Land lightly and softly on the mid-foot. Return to the start position and repeat.

Spotty dogs: A good introduction exercise for Short HIIT, this one. The coordination takes a bit of getting used to, but once mastered it's great for working all the major muscles and joints. Begin by striding forward with one foot while taking the other foot back behind the body. Don't over-stride – it need only be a short distance. Jump the foot forward and continue, on the spot, with this movement. Now you bring in the arms (here's where it gets tricky). Swing the right arm forward as the left leg strides forward and vice versa. Make the entire movement fluid and fast moving.

Mountain climbers: Assume a press-up position with hands on the floor, arms straight beneath the shoulders and legs straight out behind you. The balls of your feet should be touching the floor. Spring

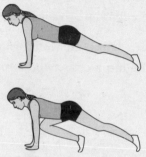

your left leg forward so that the knee touches your left elbow, return it to the start position and then spring the right leg forward so that knee touches the right elbow. Make the movement dynamic and fast, alternating left and right legs.

High knee sprints: This drill is one used by elite athletes and is perfect for intense workouts. Think of it as a sort of exaggerated running action in which you drive your

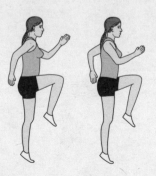

knees towards the chest. It can be done either on the spot or over a short distance of 33–50ft (10–15m). Keep a straight back and land gently on the balls of your feet, alternating left to right leg. I try to imagine running on eggs and trying not to break the shells. The movement should be light and bouncy.

Jump squats: These really work the lower body. Start in a standing position, feet shoulder width apart. Squat down by bending the knees and sticking your bottom out (imagine you are preparing to sit in a chair). Keep your back straight and your head aligned. Jump up powerfully, raising your hands above your head to aid elevation and landing as softly as you can on the balls of your feet. Repeat.

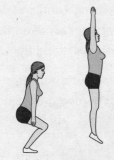

Jumping jacks: Another old-fashioned fat burner that will really send your metabolism soaring. Begin with feet together and arms at your sides. Flex the knees slightly to prepare for the movement and then jump both feet outwards, simultaneously raising the arms to form an X shape with your body. Jump the feet straight back to the centre starting position and repeat in quick succession. Make sure you keep your back straight and head up. No twisting or turning as it will cause injury.

Squat thrusts: You really notice your heart rate soaring when you do a Short HIIT session with these old favourites. Great for toning the legs, too. Start in a press-up position with palms of the

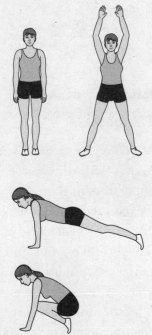

hands on the floor beneath the shoulders and legs outstretched behind you. Jump both legs forward towards the chest in a powerful movement, bending them as much as you can at the knees and raising your hands off the floor so that only fingertips are touching. Return hands and legs to the start position and repeat.

Indoor cycle sprints: In theory, you can perform these sprints on an outdoor bike, but exercise physiologists recommend sticking

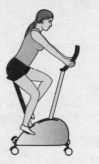

to indoor bikes as they allow you to change resistance quickly, which is what you need for this super-short session. Key here is speed – you need to push as hard as you can for the short bursts, more so than you would on a cardio or Long HIIT cycle. It's tougher than it sounds.

WEIGHT BURNERS
The basics

As you've already seen, weights are of utmost importance for an Ageless Body. However, everything you thought you knew about lifting them might well be wrong. What we should be doing to get the most out of our muscles is slowing down. In sharp contrast to the trend for endless, fast repetitions of light weights popularized by the likes of Tracy Anderson, who trains Cameron Diaz and Gwyneth Paltrow, science-backed theories advocate winding down the rate at which we lift weights to make more speedy progress.

We are not talking snail pace here, but pushing a weight to the end point in around 1–2 seconds and lowering back down to the start point in 4–5 seconds. Some advocate an even slower movement, taking 10 seconds to lift and 10 to lower the weight. It's harder than it sounds. There is a tipping point at which your quivering muscles seem unable to perform another repetition but when it is important to push on.

In the US, high profile trainers like Adam Zickerman, whose clients include A-listers such as Sharon Stone and Uma Thurman, rave about slower weights, claiming they achieve results faster than hammering away in the gym. But how? By slowing down, the muscles are forced to work harder, unable to rely on momentum to propel movement. As a consequence they get much more tired by decreasing acceleration so that the intensity is prolonged.

There's plenty of evidence that it works and not just from the Ageless Bodies of those practising it. Three decades ago a group of exercise physiologists at the University of Florida, led by Ken Hutchins, discovered that the super-slow approach was beneficial to women with osteoporosis and that it helped to maintain bone mass better than other workouts [81]. Elite athletes tend to favour the longer, steadier approach to resistance training and a study published in the *Journal of Sports Medicine and Physical Fitness* showed that short sessions of slower, intense weight training produced 50 per cent greater improvements in muscle tone than longer, quicker workouts using lighter weights [82].

I find it useful to position a stopwatch or clock in front of my nose. Better still, a metronome if you really want to slow down your exercise. There are plenty around. Try the exercise-specific Seiko Quartz Metronome or a free app such as Tempo SlowMo.

Triceps overhead extension: Develops muscle tone in the pesky backs of the arms that are so prone to hanging flesh. You need one

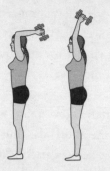

dumbbell for the exercise. Hold it at one end with both hands while standing upright, feet shoulder width apart. Keep head up, back straight and lift the dumbbell above your head by straightening and lifting your arms. Hold the dumbbell at the top so that the weight drops towards your back. Keeping arms close to your head and with elbows in a fixed position for the entire move, lower the dumbbell behind your head by bending the elbows. Continue until elbows are bent to about 45 degrees and then slowly raise the weight back up above your head. Repeat.

Shoulder press: You can do this exercise sitting on a chair or the end of a bench or standing up, feet shoulder width apart. If you

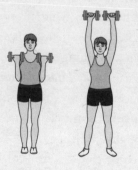

do stand up, make sure you keep a bit of flexion in the knees and that your back remains straight. Engage the abdominal muscles for trunk support and hold a dumbbell in each hand. Bend your elbows and raise the weights so that they are just above shoulder level, palms facing forward (start position). In a slow, controlled movement, push the weights overhead simultaneously. Lower back down to the start position and repeat the movement.

Single arm fly: Hold a dumbbell in the right hand. Lie on a bench if you have one, or on the floor if not, placing feet flat on the floor and knees bent. Extend the right arm out to the side, keeping the elbow slightly bent. Place your left hand on your left hip for support. Bring the weight above the chest and then out to the side again. Repeat for the set number of repetitions before changing sides.

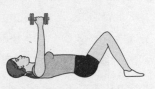

Lateral raise: This gives great shape to the upper shoulders. Stand with feet shoulder width apart, holding a dumbbell in each hand.

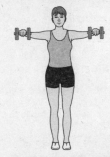

Arms should be by your sides and palms facing the body. Contract your abdominal muscles to stay strong in the trunk and then raise the weights to the sides, lifting upwards with straight arms (elbows not locked) until your arms are parallel to the floor. Lower back down and repeat.

Arnold press: Another shoulder exercise (named after Arnold Schwarzenegger – although don't be concerned that you'll achieve anything like his level of bulk). Sit on a dining chair or the end of a bench and hold a dumbbell in each hand. Feet should be flat on the floor, back straight and head facing forward. Position the dumbbells so that palms are facing upwards and the weights are at shoulder height, keeping

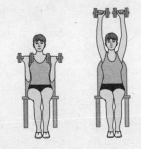

elbows close to the body. From there, open the arms to the sides with elbows bent at 90 degrees and upper arms almost parallel to the floor. Press the weights up and over the head. Then lower the weights back down to the mid-position (wide) and then the start position (close to the body). Repeat.

Reverse fly: Great for correcting poor posture. Hold a dumbbell in each hand and stand with feet shoulder width apart. Lean

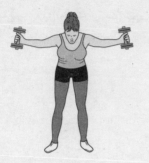

forward from the hips to an angle of around 45 degrees, keeping your back straight and your head aligned. From this position allow the weights to hang from your arms below your body. Simultaneously raise the arms out to the sides until they are level with the shoulders. Don't lock the elbows. Return to the start position and repeat.

Triceps kick back: Get rid of bingo wings with this move. It also tones the tummy. Hold a dumbbell in each hand, palms facing

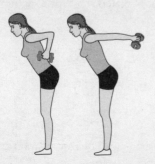

inwards, and stand with feet shoulder width apart. Feet should be planted firmly on the floor. Bend forward from the hips and bend the elbows, keeping upper arms tucked into the sides of your trunk. Keeping those upper arms in position, slowly extend the lower arms behind you until your arms form a straight position without completely locking the elbows. Bring the lower arms back in by bending the elbows and repeat.

Weighted calf raise: The calves are among the most neglected muscles in the average workout regimen. Not this one. This move really helps to create tone in the muscle and to avoid the dreaded cankle appearance. Hold a dumbbell in each hand and stand straight, feet shoulder width apart, looking ahead. Without leaning forward (you really don't want to wobble at all), slowly raise up on to the balls of your feet, feeling those calf muscles working to 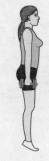 push you upwards. Hold for a second before lowering slowly back down. Repeat.

Weighted side bend: Oh, for the trim waist of your thirties. This is one step closer to achieving it. This is a tough move, so try it with a single dumbbell first to get the technique mastered. Stand upright, feet shoulder width apart and abdominal muscles engaged. Hold a dumbbell in each hand (or a single weight with both hands) above your head with arms straight (but elbows not locked). If using two weights, the ends of the weights should be an inch 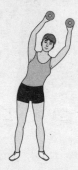 or so apart, not touching. Hold that position and flex sideways from the waist towards the left as far as you can without feeling strain or discomfort. Return to the start position and repeat to the right. Repeat.

Bicep curl: This works for shapely upper arms, toning the muscles at the front of the limbs. Hold a dumbbell in each hand and stand

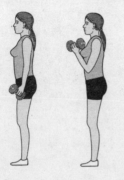

with feet shoulder width apart. Engage your abdominal muscles and raise the weights by bending your elbows, palms facing the body. Curl the weights up towards the shoulders, keeping elbows close to your trunk. When the weights reach chest level, slowly uncurl back down.

Upright row: Great for toning the fronts of the arms and the shoulders. Hold a weight in each hand and stand with feet shoulder

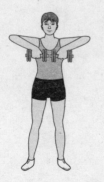

width apart, palms facing inwards. Keep your back straight and your eyes looking straight ahead. Leading with your elbows, lift the dumbbells upwards to chest level. You should reach the point where upper arms are about level with the shoulders. Return to the start position and repeat.

Bent over row: This is an all-round upper body strengthener that really helps to create a sexy back. Hold a dumbbell in each hand and stand with feet hip width apart. Bend your knees and then flex forward from the hips, keeping your back straight and head aligned.

Allow the weights to travel down towards the floor, palms facing the body. Engage your abdominal muscles and simultaneously lift both weights upwards towards the ribcage by bending the elbows. Keep going until your arms are bent at a 45 degree angle. Lower the weight back down and repeat.

Woodchopper: You need one dumbbell for this waist-trimming move. Hold the weight in both hands and stand with feet shoulder width apart. Flex your knees slightly and raise the dumbbell to your right shoulder level. In a slow, controlled movement, move the weight across the front of your body and towards the left of your body as you would if you were chopping a piece of wood. The weight should move just past your left hip. Return to the start position and repeat for the set number of repetitions before switching sides.

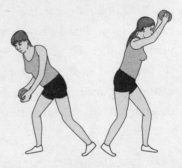

CALISTHENICS

The basics

Given that you are of an age appropriate to the target audience of this book, then you might well remember calisthenics from the first time around. In the 1980s it was a trend for the ladies-in-legwarmers brigade who vainly attempted to spot-reduce fat from various parts of the body. Unsuccessfully, I might add. It is back in fashion, but, as you might imagine, with more scientific backing and requiring considerably more gusto.

Calisthenics is an umbrella term for any move that uses the body weight for resistance – there are no weights, kettle bells, treadmills or any of the other trendy gym accessories involved. What is required is effort and in bucket loads. Far from the gentle stretching and toning approach with which it was once associated, the born-again version can be anything from a fast-paced and pant-provoking routine of every conceivable version of push-up, jumping jack and squat thrust, to the repetitions of the kind of body-lifting moves that leave you quivering like jelly.

Celebrities love it, not least because it is so portable it can be practised in a hotel room anywhere. Helen Mirren does a form of calisthenics with the 12-minute Royal Canadian Air Force exercise plan that includes stretches, push-ups, sit-ups and on-the-spot running. And for further proof that it can produce dramatic results in the over forties, look no further than the bodies of Jennifer Aniston and Madonna, both of whom use elements of it in their workouts.

Push-up: The traditional push-up continually rates as the best all-round exercise you can do on a regular basis. There are varieties (moving your arms in and out, altering the space between the hands),

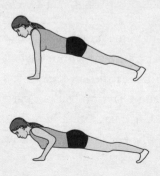

but try to perfect the original before moving on to more advanced manoeuvres. Lie face down on the floor with legs together and the palms of your hands on the floor just beneath the shoulders. Extend legs behind you, supporting them with the balls of your feet. Push the hands into the floor and straighten your arms to raise yourself up. Engage your abdominal muscles to help you achieve this. Don't completely lock the elbows at the top of the move, and do try to keep your body in a straight line. Lower yourself back down by bending the elbows to around 45 degrees, and repeat. Beginners can try the same upper body movement but with knees on the floor.

Squats: If there's an ultimate exercise for the lower body, it is this one. No regimen should be without the super-squat. Yes, it's tough, but the results more than offset the effort involved. Stand with feet shoulder width apart and firmly planted on the ground. Either cross your hands at shoulder level or position arms in front of you for balance. Then flex from the hips, keeping weight in your heels to prevent you toppling over. Stick out your bottom as if you are preparing to sit in a chair. Keep lowering until your knees are bent at almost 90 degrees, making sure your back remains straight and your head is aligned. Slowly raise back up to the start position. Repeat.

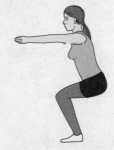

Sumo squats: A variation on the traditional squat that tweaks the position to alter the muscles worked. To do it, stand with feet slightly wider than hip width apart, knees and toes pointing out at a 45 degree angle. Again, you can position your hands either crossed at shoulder height or in front of you for balance. Bend your knees and lower your

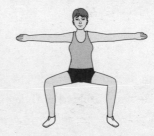

233

bottom as if preparing to sit, keeping heels rooted to the ground for good balance. Make sure the back is straight and eyes are looking forward throughout. Continue until knees are at 45 degrees, then slowly return to the start position. Repeat.

Walking lunge: I defy anyone not to ache after doing these for the first time. Persevere though as they are among the best leg and buttock toners around. The walking lunge also requires balance and core strength. An all-round super-toner. Start with feet shoulder width apart and hands by your sides. Raise your left leg and bend

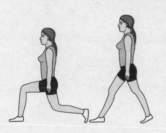

the knee to 90 degrees before taking a stride forward into a lunge with it. Keep your left knee over your left foot, not in front of it, back straight and eyes looking straight ahead. Repeat with the right foot taking alternate steps for the set number of repetitions.

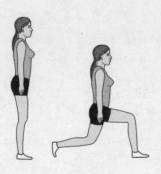

Alternate lunge: If you don't have the space for walking lunges inside, you may prefer the alternate leg lunge which can be done more or less on the spot. Again, step forward with the left leg from a standing position into a lunge, keeping your back straight and eyes ahead. Push back up to the start position and repeat with the right leg.

Single leg body lift: The first time I tried this I wondered why I had ever bothered with leg machines at the gym at all. It is super-effective at strengthening the leg and core muscles (brought into action as you stabilize the body). You'll need a bench or sturdy chair. Start by lying on your back on the floor, both feet on the bench and bottom fairly close to it. Take off your left foot and flex it towards the ceiling. Placing your arms on the floor beside you, palms down, raise 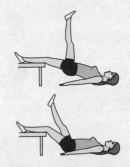 your pelvis off the floor using the muscles in your right leg as well as those in the core to power the move. Continue until your hips are in line with your shoulders. Lower back down to the start position, repeating for the set number of repetitions before switching legs.

Wall squats: An old-fashioned favourite, perfect for doing in front of the TV. Don't be fooled into thinking it's as easy as it looks.

Stand upright with your back against a wall. Slide your back down the wall as you walk your feet forward in small, shuffling steps. Keep going until your thighs are parallel to the floor. Press your heels into the floor and make sure your ankles are beneath your knees. Keep your head 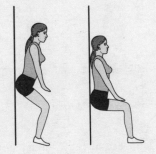 up and eyes looking forward. I find it's best to place my hands on my thighs, but position them where you feel comfortable. You'll need to engage your core muscles as you 'sit' there, so this move works the entire lower body. Hold for the recommended duration.

Step-up: Another simple exercise that builds strength, power and tone in the buttock muscles and the backs of the legs. You will

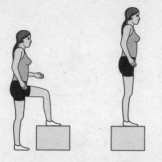

need a sturdy bench, box or chair. Stand next to the platform and place your left foot on the top surface so that your knee bends at around 90 degrees (it needn't be exact but too much or too little of an angle will produce detrimental results). Push up through the heels of your left foot to raise your body and place your right foot on the surface next to your left. Step down again with your left foot. Repeat the set number of repetitions on your left leg before switching to the right.

Chair dips: Another arm toning exercise that requires no accessories other than a bench or chair. It really is effective at toning

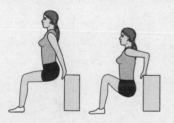

the triceps at the backs of the arms. Position your hands on the edge of the bench, palms down and fingers facing your body. Feet should be flat on the floor and far enough away from the bench to allow you to drop your body down by bending your arms. Lower your body until your arms are at right angles and your upper arm parallel to the floor. Keep your back straight and eyes looking straight ahead. Push your body back up to the start position using your arms and pushing your heels into the floor. Complete the set number of repetitions.

Lateral lunges: Here's one I love for its ability to target the inner thigh, a tricky to reach body part, as well as the buttocks. Start with legs wide apart, back straight and eyes looking forward. Allow your arms to hang by your sides. Bend your left knee, aiming to get the left thigh almost parallel to the floor. Your right leg remains in a straight position (without completely locking the knee). Press the left foot into the floor to return to the start position and repeat the movement on the other side. Alternate for the set number of repetitions.

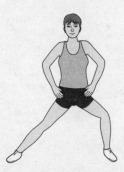

ABS EXERCISES

Much of what we thought we knew about toning abdominal muscles has been overthrown in recent years. Endless sit-ups and crunches are out in favour of a variety of abs exercises designed to work the musculature that wraps around and supports our trunk in its entirety. What's more, it is more than possible to flaunt a six-pack style-middle well into your forties and beyond. It's also known, however, that abs can't be spot-toned, that is we shouldn't work on them exclusively. Cardio, squats and lunges are among the best exercises for a lean middle because they are great calorie burners, reducing all-over body fat to reveal muscles beneath. Our abs sessions have a mix of the most effective moves, guaranteed to get your midriff toned even if you can't quite bring yourself to wear a crop top.

Crunch: Although maligned as the six-pack solution in recent years, the crunch is still an important part of an overall midriff-toning regimen. To do it, lie on your back, hands positioned lightly at the sides of your head. Place feet flat on the floor, knees bent and curl

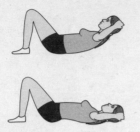

your upper body towards them. Key here is not to 'sit up' but to keep the lower back on the floor. Your chin should be tucked in and head held in position. Lower back down and repeat for the set number of repetitions.

Superman: My feeling is that it should be renamed the Superwoman for its ability to work the abs, bottom and lower back.

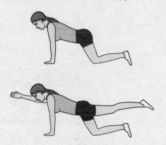

Start on your hands and knees with knees directly beneath your hips and hands beneath your shoulders. Palms should be flat on the floor and fingers facing forwards. In a controlled movement, raise your right arm and left leg, extending each forward and backward accordingly. If it's easier, extend your arm first before lifting your leg. Hold the position for the set amount of time before returning to the start position and switching sides.

Plank: Lie face down with hands positioned palms down, facing forwards and beneath your shoulders. Elbows and feet should be on

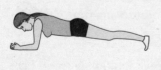

the floor. Raise your body onto your forearms (with elbows bent to 90 degrees) and feet, keeping your back, head and legs in a straight line. Hold the position for the recommended time.

Oblique crunch: The sideways version of the crunch that hits the waist and love handles. Lie on your back on the floor, hands positioned lightly at the sides of your head. Bring your feet close to your buttocks, feet flat on the floor. Using your abdominal muscles, twist your right elbow to your left knee, raising your shoulders off the floor as you do so. Lower back down and repeat on the other side. Repeat for the set number of repetitions.

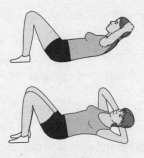

V-sits: These are tough but really do get results. You use the front abdominal muscles as well as the obliques at the sides for balance. Lie on your back on the floor, hands positioned lightly at the sides of your head and legs outstretched. Simultaneously raise your upper and lower body to form a 'V' position in which you balance on your buttocks. Knees can be slightly bent. Lower back down in a controlled way, really engaging your core muscles for support. Repeat for the set number of repetitions.

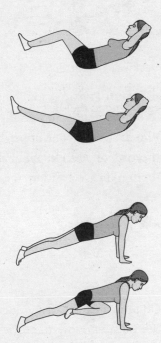

Knee crossovers: A dynamic abs-toning move that really helps develop stability in the area. Start in a press-up position, supported by the feet and with hands beneath the shoulders, fingers forward. Engage your abs to hold the trunk in position and then raise your left knee towards your right arm. Your back should not 'bend' or twist' and you need to return to the start position if this happens. Repeat by raising your right knee to your left arm and alternate in this way for the set number of repetitions.

Side plank: A tough adaptation of the traditional plank that is well worth conquering for its strengthening benefits. Start by lying on your right side and lift your body, supporting yourself on your right forearm and feet. Make sure your body is straight and forms a

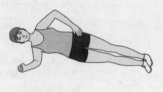

diagonal line from feet to head. Keep your head in line with your body. Hold the position for the required amount of time before repeating on the other side. As you get fitter, try performing side plank raises by dropping and raising your hips to the floor from this position.

Russian Twist: A tough move, but you'll be thankful you endured it for the results. Sit upright on the floor, knees bent and feet flat on the mat. Lean your upper body back a little and raise your hands in front of you, clasping hands together lightly. Balancing on your bottom in a V position, raise your legs off the floor by a few inches,

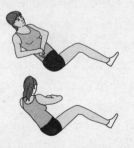

knees slightly bent. Keep your head up and eyes forward. Still balancing, lower your clasped hands towards the right of your body. Return to the start position and repeat on the left side. Repeat the entire movement for the set number of repetitions.

CHAPTER ELEVEN

HOW TO KEEP GOING

Most new diet and exercise regimens begin with a flurry of optimism and excitement. It's not difficult to launch yourself into an overhaul of your lifestyle habits when so much is at stake. Maintaining the momentum is trickier and there will inevitably be times when you feel your healthy approach is beginning to come unstuck. What then?

Given that we have experienced the ebb and flow ourselves (we are no saints), we are in an ideal position to steer you along the straight and narrow, to help you build on the good foundations that have been laid down.

EATING

Our four-week eating plan is designed to be adaptable and flexible. You might find that you need to stick to it more or less to the letter as you embark on phase 1 of the exercise plan, but by the time you get started on phase 2 of the workouts you will almost certainly become more adept at knowing what and when to eat. At this point you can experiment more with ingredients and meal swaps.

By phase 3 of the exercise plan you might want to add in some of your own favourite healthy ingredients and meals. If that's the case, stick to 1400–1600 calories a day and ensure you don't break the 4-hour fast rule. You'll find that this, along with breakfast skipping and the one healthy carb-based meal a day, becomes a way of life. Which is precisely what we hoped would happen. While we don't encourage setting a target weight (an Ageless Body is more about how you feel and look rather than numbers on the scales), we appreciate that some of you find it helps with motivation. That's fine, just don't get fixated by fluctuations in weight. And keep it up, even when goals are met. The Ageless Body plan is not just a passing fad, it is for life. You'll feel all the better for it.

EXERCISE

By the end of phase 1 of our exercise plan, your body will be transformed. If you stick with the workouts right the way through, you will barely resemble the person you were at the start. But what then? In order for exercise to be effective, it must be consistent and progressive. All of the scientific evidence supports our approach of four workouts a week past the age of 40, so there's absolutely no need to increase the number of sessions beyond that.

Towards the end of the total 12-week exercise plan, we have slotted in some additional gentle cardio sessions which are purely optional. If you choose to add some of these, keep them to 45 minutes and under, and don't turn them into temp (speedy) or interval workouts. With the Short and Long HIIT training, your aim should be to achieve more in the same time frame or to slightly increase the number of minutes you spend exercising. Be careful not to increase the total amount you are doing by more than 10 per cent a week.

If you are motivated by trying new things or like exercising in groups, then there's plenty out there to light your fire and help with rejuvenation of body and mind. Personally, I dip in and out of as many of these as takes my fancy, maintaining my four weekly sessions as my bedrock. Here are five of my favourites:

Hatha yoga: Good for stress and boosting brain function. Researchers at the University of Illinois studied 108 adults between the ages of 55 and 79, 61 of whom attended hatha yoga classes. At the end of eight weeks, the group that did yoga three times a week performed better on cognitive tests than it had before the start of the trial [83]. British Wheel of Yoga has a list of classes (bwy.org.uk).

Assisted stretching: Ever since I had a session of assisted stretching with Suzanne Waterworth, one of the UK's leading practitioners, I have been a firm fan of this. The stretches are deep and controlled and your body is pushed and pulled through a range of movement by a therapist. You leave feeling that you really have rolled back the years. Thoroughly recommended. You can try it at: triyoga.co.uk; Suzanne Waterworth at www.revive-stretching.com; Burn 360 at virginactive.com; and Dalton Wong at twentytwotraining.com.

Rev5 (rev5.co.uk): Slow weight training has been a trend in the US for a while (Sharon Stone and Uma Thurman are fans), but this company, headed by Dr Tahir Masood who became convinced of the health benefits after using the approach with diabetes patients, is rolling out classes in the UK. Its premise is that lifting heavy weights at a snail's pace for just 15 minutes once a week will build unparalleled levels of muscle strength and tone. All in your lunch hour.

Barre workouts: Charlize Theron and Madonna have long taken ballet classes and Carine Roitfeld, the smouldering former editor of French *Vogue*, attributes her ability to do the splits at 58 to her private ballet classes in her Parisian flat.

Now more and more ordinary women feel a call to the barre with a range of classes that incorporate elements of ballet's limb-lengthening and toning moves. Everywhere from Equinox gym, where members can try Barre Burn, to beginner classes run by the English National Ballet and the Central School of Ballet and bespoke studios such as Ballet-tone and Barretoned, which combine resistance training and dance, are jumping on the ballet bandwagon.

Treadmill: I'm a confirmed outdoor runner, so I was surprised to find that I thoroughly enjoyed the new wave of treadmill classes that are sweeping gyms. In New York, short, sharp running sessions on a belt are hugely fashionable with venues like the Mile High Run Club and Run, both dedicated treadmill running studios, offering sessions on state-of-the-art Woodway treadmills – £7000 machines with belt surfaces like tank treads that are supposed to mimic the feel of trail running and, according to the manufacturers, are kinder to joints and connective tissues. In the UK, Equinox and Virgin Active have their own versions that are very much like the HIIT sessions we advocate in this book.

FIVE WAYS TO THINK YOURSELF TO AN AGELESS BODY

It's all very well having great intentions, but if your mind's not willing then your body almost certainly isn't either. Psychology plays a huge role in the success of any new lifestyle change and it can sometimes feel like an uphill struggle for even the most diligent healthy eater and exerciser. Researchers have pored over the reasons why we are sometimes stumped in our attempts to stay on the well-being straight and narrow. And the most likely culprit when it comes to diverting from the course is attitude.

Some psychologists have hinted that women are genetically programmed to feel the pressure to stay in shape more than men and that motivation to exercise differs between the sexes. In one study by psychologists at the University of Birmingham's School of Sport and Exercise Science, Dr Elizabeth Loughren surveyed almost 1000 first-time marathon runners aged 18–72 and found that whereas most men were putting themselves through the gruelling course of 26 miles because it provided a personal challenge, most women were doing it to improve their appearance or lose weight [84].

Another survey by the American College of Sports Medicine showed that, for most women, thinness was the prime motivator for working out whereas men wanted to improve their strength [85]. Not that it's all doom and gloom. Just as we can train our bodies to become more efficient, so we can coax our minds to become more focused and to respond better to motivational triggers. Here are five ways you can help to keep attention (and motivation) focused:

♥ Set exercise goals that are specific, measurable and realistic with distinct time boundaries, not one big goal that can be overwhelming. For example, the goal might be 'I want to run a 5km fun run in two months' time'. Intersperse smaller goals en route to your main aim – you will run three times a week to achieve that, and will run 1 mile (2km) without stopping by the end of next week.

♥ Write things down. Pin your main goal up on a noticeboard or on the fridge. Detail all of your exercise in a diary so that on tougher days you can look back and see how far you have come.

♥ Be self-critical. Regularly re-assess your goals to make sure you are on track. If you fail to meet a particular target, don't get disheartened – re-adjust your expectations until you meet them.

♥ Don't set weekly or monthly weight goals to be reached by certain dates. The likelihood is you will be disappointed and lack the motivation to continue.

♥ Don't judge your progress solely on appearance or pounds lost. Focus instead on how many weights you have lifted, workouts you have completed or how far you have come.

THE 10 COMMANDMENTS OF AN AGELESS BODY FOR LIFE

1. *Don't eat when you are not hungry*: If there's one thing we hope you have learned while following the plan it is that hunger is a positive thing. It is a signal that your body is working well and is certainly not something that should be feared or, indeed, satiated at every opportunity. The French have this sussed, rarely snacking between meals so that they arrive for a meal with a good appetite. We don't want you to feel starving by any means, just pleasantly hungry (that's not a contradiction in terms, you will soon discover). Likewise, learn to stop eating before you are stuffed. Reconnecting with our hunger cues is vital in terms of weight loss, helping to prevent the panicked rush to the biscuit tin.

2. *Plan your meals to suit you, nobody else*: Our overbearing belief is that all meals are equal – breakfast is not nutritionally superior to brunch, just as dinner doesn't usurp supper in the nutrient stakes. So, if you prefer not to eat at a certain time of the day, don't feel guilty about it. Too much emphasis has been placed on the importance of starting the day on a full stomach when, in fact, there is scant evidence to support the practice. Both of us find that we tend to eat more throughout the day (and studies confirm we are not alone), so experiment and work out for yourself when your body prefers to eat.

3. Stick to four workouts a week: Less is more as you get older (although you almost certainly need to up the pace). We have based our four-days-a-week workout plan not only on personal trials, but on science. There's plenty of evidence that this amount of hardcore effort is all that's required as you get older, provided you intersperse with general activity as well. One trial at the University of Alabama looked at a group of previously sedentary older women who were split into groups and asked to follow different regimens for 16 weeks. At the end of the trial they found participants on a four-days-a-week plan burned more calories per session than those on a six-day programme [86].

4. Lift weights: If there's an element of exercise everyone should introduce as they get older, it's this one. As we've seen, regular weight training preserves muscle mass, strengthens bones and leaves you looking leaner and longer. It also triggers tremendous 'afterburn' of calories. A study in *The Journal of Strength and Conditioning Research* found that women who did an hour of strength training burned about 100 calories more the day following their workout than they did when they didn't lift weights [87]. It doesn't sound much, but over the course of a year the difference to your energy usage will be considerable. Not to mention your appearance.

5. Base only one meal a day around carbs: Our advice flies in the face of government recommendations, but we believe those recommendation to be hopelessly outdated. Our suggestion is that only one meal a day is based on carbs. We certainly don't suggest you cut down too drastically on carbs or, as on some fashionable diets, eliminate them. With just one meal a day based on carbs in the form of whole grains, you will obtain carbs from dairy, fruit or starchy vegetables at other times. Protein should be eaten at every meal because it helps you to feel full quickly and for longer, so you don't feel the need to snack.

6. Eat fruit: Shunned for its sugar content, we are advocates of fruit, although not as an in-between snack (heaven forbid), with a bowl of berries on your desk to nibble on, paleo-style, all day. An issue for adults is the high GI content of many fruits. But fruits are rich in nutrients and fibre and adding them to savoury meals instantly lowers their GI and the adverse shock they have on your blood sugar levels. We agree that sugar-laden, processed foods should be sidelined, but fruits are firm favourites of ours and we urge you not to ditch them.

7. Don't fuel (or refuel) your workouts: Unless you are an elite athlete who needs a precise and measured input of fuel (which, let's face it, is unlikely at our age), then it's a huge misconception that you need to fuel and re-fuel for a workout. Cast aside all notion of energy bars and sugar-laden sports drinks being essential to replacing what's lost when you exercise. Don't head for a smoothie and a bran muffin when you finish just because you feel your glycogen levels have plummeted. You need to eat and drink, yes, but our nutrition plan will more than suffice.

8. Eat fat: We have been told to keep saturated animal fats to a minimum and to increase our intake of so-called healthy polyun-saturated fats – such as omega-3 or omega-6, found in oily fish and plant-based foods – to reduce heart disease. However, the guidance is now under review after a major British Heart Foundation-funded study at the University of Cambridge concluded that there was insufficient evidence to back up such recommendations [88]. So what is the current advice? Eat a range of healthy fats, including the saturated variety in the form of lean meat and some dairy, along with other fats from nuts, avocados, oily fish and seeds.

9. Stick to a 4-Hour fast: Your body was not designed to be drip-fed with calories throughout the day. It needs a break from constant consumption of energy in order to re-set itself to optimal health mode. A 4 or more hour break between meals is not unnatural – it is what our physiological make-up craves. And remember that studies show that a larger meal eaten in one go is also more wasteful of calories than if the same foods were eaten as a sequence of snacks. In other words, you'll retain more of the calories eaten as snacks than you would eaten as one meal. Researchers at the University of Kansas Medical Center found that the more often you eat, the less likely you are to feel full [89]. In fact, constant snacking makes you think you are more hungry when you really are not – leading to higher caloric intake and eventual weight gain. We push eating larger meals and feeling more satisfied.

10. Enjoy your body, enjoy your life: Researchers at the University of Warwick have found that the older you get the happier you become. A blip in the mid-forties aside (a time when, apparently, you are most likely to hit a depressive dip – we are not listening), Professor Andrew Oswald and his team showed that happiness levels follow a U-shape curve rising as people move into their late forties onwards [90]. And, ultimately, your state of mind is perhaps your most powerful ally. University College London researchers conducted a study of 10,000 English people that suggested future disability and poor health could be predicted by the state of a person's mind. Those who enjoyed life the most were three times more likely to live a little longer than those who enjoyed it the least [91]. A happy ageing body is a healthy one.

CHAPTER TWELVE

TROUBLESHOOTER

All is going swimmingly, only for you to discover that your good intentions hit a hurdle. We try to answer some of the most common queries about the Ageless Body plan below:

What if I get hungry?

Don't panic. It's normal to feel a certain amount of hunger when you are trying to lose weight, and plans that promise you won't experience it at all simply don't work. You need to get used to feeling hungry – that's the niggling background hunger, not the ravenous type that throws you completely off kilter. Prior to the snacking culture, this was something our grandparents and parents experienced daily. We've forgotten what it's like to have a rumbling stomach. Just be sure that your body will adapt quickly and you'll be able to cope better after a few weeks. Remember, if you are feeling hungry your body will be using up its fat stores. If on the other hand you feel you simply must eat, have yogurt and berries, oatcakes with peanut butter or hummus.

<u>I'm concerned that high intensity exercise is dangerous as I've heard some horror stories. Are they true?</u>

No form of physical activity can be entirely risk-free. But the risks of a sedentary lifestyle far outweigh any dangers associated with regularly exercising. In truth, our bodies are cleverly programmed to send warning signals when we are pushing ourselves hard. They operate within their own boundaries and only in very rare and extreme cases are we able to push ourselves into the danger zone. We instinctively know when we have reached the upper limits of our own fitness levels. Much of the recent adverse publicity surrounding HIIT stemmed from claims made by the BBC broadcaster Andrew Marr that a stroke he suffered was linked to an intense workout on the rowing machine. However, Marr had suffered from previous silent strokes, so an underlying problem existed. And the Stroke Association charity clearly states that exercise is one of the best means of preventing the condition, rather than causing it. Numerous studies have looked specifically at the effects of HIIT on the heart. In one Norwegian study of patients considered at high risk of a heart attack who were asked to follow a HIIT programme or a gentle aerobics regimen, the researchers concluded: 'Considering the significant cardiovascular adaptations associated with high intensity exercise, such exercise should be considered among patients with coronary artery disease' [92]. That said, it is always recommended to consult a medical professional if you have had heart disease in the past, are considered at high risk of getting it or if there is a family history of the condition.

<u>My weight loss has plateaued – why?</u>

Weight loss is always exponential so the more you have to lose the faster it will come off at the beginning. When you start to plateau is the time to step up both your exercise and your incidental daily activity. You'll be feeling fitter the further you get into the plan, so increase the effort you put into your exercise and pick up the general daily activity in your life – walk or cycle everywhere, spend more time on your feet (on trains or buses), stand when you are chatting to friends, shop instead of internet order; it will all add up. It should be enough to make a difference without cutting down on food – you need enough food for good nutrition.

<u>I want to increase my general daily activity. Will a fitness tracker help?</u>

Fitness trackers are data-collectors which keep tally of every step stepped and every calorie burnt – whether while exercising or doing the housework – and have become hugely popular among adults: if it's not a Jawbone UP or a Nike+ FuelBand SE then it's a Misfit Shine device or a Garmin Vivofit. My psychologist friend tells me that they have their place as a motivational tool: people move more because they are wearing them. But don't rely on them for 100 per cent accuracy. When a team at Iowa State University tested the accuracy of eight popular fitness trackers against lab equipment that accurately measures energy expenditure, they found that some overestimated calorie burn by a massive 23 per cent [93].

<u>What about alcohol – is it allowed?</u>

Alcohol has few nutritional benefits so if you are not bothered about it and won't miss it, cut it out. However for some (myself included) it is the treat I look forward to and I'd be miserable without a glass of wine. In which case, choose your moments carefully. There are certain rules: don't drink if it will interfere with your workouts or if it will lead to a binge-drinking episode, and don't exceed the weekly recommended maximum for women of 14 units (a unit being the equivalent of a small glass of wine).

I feel incredibly stiff and heavy-legged after some of the high intensity workouts. What can be done?

This is caused by Delayed Onset Muscle Soreness (or DOMS). It's down to a natural process that occurs after vigorous exercise. Tiny tears in muscle fibres lead to an immune reaction – inflammation – as the body gets to work repairing the injured cells. It's perfectly normal and affects everyone from beginners through to elite athletes. Scientific studies have come up with all sorts of solutions to DOMS including tart cherry juice, caffeine, watermelon juice and the dreaded ice baths. Massage can help as it is thought to reduce the production of compounds called cytokines, which play a critical role in inflammation. However, the only proven remedy is rest. That's partly why we have allocated three rest days a week on the Ageless Body plan. However, if it really isn't enough, then cut your intense sessions to three a week for the first few weeks, replacing the fourth workout with some gentle cardio. The good news is that DOMS gets better the more exercise you do, whatever your age. Researchers at Ohio State University proved this to be the case in a study on ageing racehorses and confirmed that humans adapt to regular exercise in the same way [94].

Should I take supplements while following the plan?

In theory, we should be able to get all the nutrients we need from a balanced diet; in reality, even the most health conscious eater might not achieve this. Also, if you have upped your training significantly, your needs will increase for some nutrients. So supplements can be useful for those tricky vitamins and minerals like vitamin B2 and magnesium. You don't need to overdo it with expensive brands; a multivitamin a few times a week is fine.

Is walking the best way to increase my general activity?

Any movement is better than none, but walking tops the lot. Exercise psychologists at Edinburgh University have discovered that we cover 80 miles (129km) less a year on foot than we did a decade ago [95]. Despite recommendations that we should amass at least 10,000–12,000 steps a day through walking just to stay healthy – and even more (up to 15,000) to lose weight – most of us manage a paltry 3000–4000 a day. Increase the walking you do and the benefits will be enormous. Research reported in *The Lancet* found that adding 2000 moderately paced walking steps (or 20 minutes) a day to regular activity could help people to cut their risk of heart attacks and strokes by 8 per cent. Doing 4000 more steps (40 minutes of added walking) matches the gains obtained from taking cholesterol-lowering drugs. 'It reduces your cardiovascular risk by about 16–20 per cent, which is the equivalent of taking a statin,' said Dr Thomas Yates, of the Diabetes Research Centre at the University of Leicester [96]. 'However, a statin has side-effects and only reduces cholesterol. Walking has a much bigger range of health benefits.' A study of 6000 women aged 65 and older at the University of California found that those who covered that distance experienced a much slower decline in memory compared with those who walked less than half a mile a week [97].

Do I need to cool down after a session?

One accepted fact is that intense exercise should never be stopped abruptly – when you work out hard, the heart pumps faster and blood vessels expand to promote blood flow to the legs and feet. If you stop too suddenly, blood can start to pool in the lower limbs, causing dizziness. You should spend the last five minutes of a workout doing the same activity at a slower pace, although if it's an easy cardio day, just walking around is fine. A popular misconception is that cool-down stretches will stop muscles from becoming sore by flushing out lactic acid, the waste product of exercise. Soreness isn't caused by lactic acid, but by minor damage to muscle fibres, and stretching will have no effect. An Australian study of adults who had been asked to walk backwards on a treadmill for half an hour to cause calf-muscle stiffness found that those who did a 10-minute cool-down had no less soreness afterwards than those who did not [98].

I struggle to get a workout in some days. Can I incorporate it into my commute?

Cycling is one of the best ways to get fit and, if you are creative, there's no reason why you can't incorporate your Ageless Body workout into your commute on two wheels. Try a steady cycle and then perform ten 15-second bursts (15 seconds recovery); eight 30-second bursts (30 seconds recovery) or six 45-second bursts (45 seconds recovery). The effort should be hard and fast, a sort of eyeballs-out approach. Always cool down at the end with a

5–10-minute gentle cycle. Matt Roberts, the personal trainer, is a big fan of the biking commute. His favourite session is a warm-up by cycling at a steady pace for 5 minutes before picking up the intensity and pedalling hard until you reach the first set of traffic lights or a roundabout. Take a breather until you need to go again and repeat at the same high intensity. I also like to race to catch up fellow cyclists; you can develop your own speed games like these. Maybe ride fast for five lampposts or 15 parked cars, recover, then repeat. Use your journey well.

<u>What happens if I cheat?</u>
Everybody cheats on a diet occasionally. Rather than let it get to you, gnawing away at your conscience, schedule in your cheat day be it a wedding, a party or just a BBQ with friends. But pick and choose and don't schedule in more than one a week. That way you can enjoy and move on the next day without feeling bad.

About the authors

Peta Bee is a health and fitness journalist who writes for *The Times, Sunday Times* and *Irish Examiner* and is performance editor for *Athletics Weekly* and *Running Monthly* magazines. With degrees

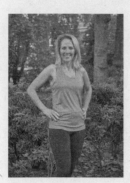

in Sports Science and Nutrition, Peta likes to probe the evidence behind the latest fads and trends, and her work has won her numerous awards including the Medical Journalists' Association's Freelancer of the Year (twice). She has appeared widely on television and radio and is the author/co-author of seven books, including *Fast Exercise*, the 2014 bestseller co-written with Dr Michael Mosley, and *The Ice Diet*.

Dr Sarah Schenker is a registered dietitian and nutritionist with a PhD in Nutrition and an Accreditation in Sports Dietetics. She is a member of

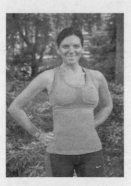

the British Dietetic Association, The Nutrition Society and The Association for Nutrition. Sarah was a contributor to the bestselling *Fast Diet Recipe Book* and regularly contributes to newspapers and magazines including the *Daily Mail, Top Santé, Reveal* and *Glamour* as well as shows including *This Morning, Watchdog* and on BBC Radio. Sarah has also worked as a nutrition adviser to several Premiership football clubs.

References

1. Escentual.com (2015)
2. Tarnopolsky et al; presented at American Medical Society for Sports Medicine annual meeting 2014
3. S. R. Davis, C. Castelo-Branco, P. Chedraui, M. A. Lumsden, R. E. Nappi, D. Shah, P. Villaseca. Understanding weight gain at menopause. Climacteric, 2012; 15 (5): 419
4. Espel, E, Brownell, K, Ickovics, J et al; Stress May Cause Excess Abdominal Fat In Otherwise Slender Women. Psychometric Medicine; September/October 2000.
5. Horvath, S; DNA methylation age of human tissues and cell types. Genome Biology; 2013;14(10):R115.
6. Prima magazine survey of 1300 women; December 2010
7. Mama Mio survey by Populus; July 2012
8. Tarnopolsky et al; Endurance exercise rescues progeroid aging and induces systemic mitochondrial rejuvenation in mtDNA mutator mice. Proceedings of the National Academy of Sciences of the United States of America; vol. 108 no. 10, 4135–4140
9. Ginsberg, S et al; "Calorie-restricting diets slow aging" ScienceDaily. ScienceDaily, 17 November 2014
10. Carlson, Martin et al; Impact of Reduced Meal Frequency Without Caloric Restriction on Glucose Regulation in Healthy, Normal Weight Middle-Aged Men and Women. Metabolism; 2007 Dec; 56(12); 179-1734
11. Brandhorst et al; A Periodic Diet that Mimics Fasting Promotes Multi-System Regeneration, Enhanced Cognitive Performance, and Healthspan; Cell Metabolism Volume 22 (issue 1); July 7 2015; 86-89
12. Cindy W. Leung, Barbara A. Laraia, Belinda L. Needham, David H. Rehkopf, Nancy E. Adler, Jue Lin, Elizabeth H. Blackburn, and Elissa S. Epel. Soda and Cell Aging: Associations Between Sugar-Sweetened Beverage Consumption and Leukocyte Telomere Length in Healthy Adults From the National Health and Nutrition Examination Surveys. American Journal of Public Health: December 2014, Vol. 104, No. 12, pp. 2425-2431
13. Wisloff, U et al; A simple nonexercise model of cardiorespiratory fitness predicts long-term mortality; Med sci Sports Exercise; 2014 Jun;46(6):1159-65.
14. Francisco B. Ortega, Duck-chul Lee, Peter T. Katzmarzyk, Jonatan R. Ruiz, Xuemei Sui, Timothy S. Church, and Steven N. Blair. The intriguing metabolically healthy but obese phenotype: cardiovascular prognosis and role of fitness. European Heart Journal, 2012;
15. And 16."Quantification of biological aging in young adults," Daniel Belsky, Avshalom Caspi, et al. PNAS, July 7, 2015. DOI: 10.1073/pnas.1506264112
16. Spector et al; Epigenome-Wide Scans Identify Differentially Methylated Regions for Age and Age-Related Phenotypes in a Healthy Ageing Population; PLOS One April 19, 2012
17. Rottensteiner. Leskinen et al; Physical activity, fitness, glucose homeostasis, and brain morphology in twins. Med Sci Sports Exercise; 2015 Mar;47(3):509-18.

18. Kroenke, Candyce H.; Caan, Bette J.; Stefanick, Marcia L.; Anderson, Garnet; Brzyski, Robert; Johnson, Karen C.; LeBlanc, Erin; Lee, Cathy; La Croix, Andrea Z.; Park, Hannah Lui; Sims, Stacy T.; Vitolins, Mara; Wallace, Robert. Effects of a dietary intervention and weight change on vasomotor symptoms in the Women's Health Initiative. Menopause, 9 July 2012

19. Simkin-silverman LR et al; Lifestyle intervention can prevent weight gain during menopause: results from a 5-year randomized clinical trial. Ann. Behav. Med. 2003 Dec;26(3):212-20.

20. Wolfe RR. The underappreciated role of muscle in health and disease. Am J Clin Nutr. 2006;84:475–482.

21. Sagiv, M et al; Role of physical activity training in attenuation of height loss through aging; Gerentology; 2000 Sep-Oct;46(5):266-70.

22. Medical University of Vienna. "Strength training still advisable in older age." ScienceDaily. ScienceDaily, 3 April 2015.

23. Koli, J et al; Effects of Exercise on Patellar Cartilage in Women with Mild Knee Osteoarthritis.; Med Sci Sports Exerc; 2015 Sep;47(9):1767-74

24. Shaw, RB et al; Aging of the facial skeleton: aesthetic implications and rejuvenation strategies.; Plast.Reconstr. Surgery; 2011 Jan;127(1):374-83.

25. Gerontology. 2000 Sep-Oct;46(5):266-70. Role of physical activity training in attenuation of height loss through aging. Sagiv M1, Vogelaere PP, Soudry M, Ehrsam R.

26. http://www.meduniwien.ac.at/homepage/1/news-and-topstories/?tx_ttnews%5Btt_news%5D=5569

27. Osteoporos Int. 2006 Jan;17(1):109-18. Epub 2005 May 12. Effect of impact exercise on bone mineral density in elderly women with low BMD: a population-based randomized controlled 30-month intervention. Korpelainen R1, Keinänen-Kiukaanniemi S, Heikkinen J, Väänänen K, Korpelainen J.

28. Plast Reconstr Surg. 2007 Feb;119(2):675-81; discussion 682-3. Aging of the midface bony elements: a three-dimensional computed tomographic study. Shaw RB Jr1, Kahn DM.

29. Am J Clin Nutr. 2013 Nov;98(5):1298-308. doi: 10.3945/ajcn.113.064410. Epub 2013 Sep 4. Belief beyond the evidence: using the proposed effect of breakfast on obesity to show 2 practices that distort scientific evidence. Brown AW1, Bohan Brown MM, Allison DB.

30. The effectiveness of breakfast recommendations on weight loss: a randomized controlled trial1,2,3. Emily J Dhurandhar, John Dawson, Amy Alcorn, Lesli H Larsen, Elizabeth A Thomas, Michelle Cardel, Ashley C Bourland, Arne Astrup, Marie-Pierre St-Onge, James O Hill, Caroline M Apovian, James M Shikany, and David B Allison. AM J Clin Nutr 2014.

31. Am J Clin Nutr. 2014 Aug;100(2):539-47. doi:10.3945/ajcn.114.083402. Epub 2014 Jun 4. The causal role of breakfast in energy balance and health: a randomized controlled trial in lean adults. Betts JA1, Richardson JD1, Chowdhury EA1, Holman GD1, Tsintzas K1, Thompson D1.

32. European Society of Cardiology (ESC). "Cycling fast: Vigorous daily exercise recommended for a longer life." ScienceDaily. ScienceDaily, 18 September 2011.

33. Department of Health UK recommendations

34. O Peter Adams; The impact of brief high-intensity exercise on blood glucose levels; Diabetes Metab Syndr Obes. 2013; 6: 113–122.

35. An investigation into the relationship between age and physiological function in highly active older adults, by Pollock RD, Carter S, Velloso CP, Duggal NA, Lord JM, Lazaraus NR, Harridge SDR, The Journal of Physiology on Tuesday 6 January 2015.
36. Hamer et al; Taking up physical activity in later life and healthy ageing: the English longitudinal study of ageing; Br J Sports Med 2014;48:239-243
37. Duck-chul Lee et al; Leisure-Time Running Reduces All-Cause and Cardiovascular Mortality Risk; J Am Coll Cardiol. 2014;64(5):472-481.
38. Miller, WC; How effective are traditional dietary and exercise interventions for weight loss?; Med Sci Sports Exerc 1999 Aug;31(8):1129-34.
39. Mintel report on Fitness Industry
40. Neville Owen et al; Sedentary Behavior: Emerging Evidence for a New Health Risk; Mayo Clin Proc. 2010 Dec; 85(12): 1138–1141.
41. Diss, C and Kerwin, D; THE EFFECT OF AGE ON VETERAN ATHLETES LEG ELASTICITY; In Proceedings of XXIV International Symposium on Biomechanics in Sports, Salzburg, Austria, 464.
42. Juan Carlos Holedo et al; Effects of Aquatic and Dry Land Resistance Training Devices on Body Composition and Physical Capacity in Postmenopausal Women; J Hum Kinet. 2012 May; 32: 185–195.
43. Ferris, Lee T et al; Resistance Training Improves Sleep Quality in Older Adults a Pilot Study; J Sports Sci Med. 2005 Sep; 4(3): 354–360. Published online 2005 Sep 1.
44. Simmons et al; The Effects of Resistance Training and Walking on Functional Fitness in Advanced Old Age; J Aging Health February 2006 vol. 18 no. 1 91-105
45. Jokl, P et al; Master's performance in the New York City Marathon 1983–1999British Journal Sports Medicine; Vol. 38: pp 408-412, August 2004
46. McMaster University study presented at the American Medical Society for Sports Medicine annual conference, 2014
47. Lars Kaestner and Anna Bogdanova; Regulation of red cell life-span, erythropoiesis, senescence, and clearance; Front Physiol. 2014; 5: 269; Published online 2014 Jul 18.
48. Burn Your Slippers and Get out More, the Elderly Told; The Times; 25 May 2015.
49. Babraj, J et al; High Intensity Training Improves Health and Physical Function in Middle Aged Adults; Biology (Basel). 2014 Jun; 3(2): 333–344
50. A. H. Laursen, O. P. Kristiansen, J. L. Marott, P. Schnohr, E. Prescott. Intensity versus duration of physical activity: implications for the metabolic syndrome. A prospective cohort study. BMJ Open, 2012
51. Lingala, Fries et al; Long Distance Running and Knee Osteoarthritis A Prospective Study; Am J Prev Med. 2008 Aug. 35 (2); 133-138
52. Easton, J et al; Personality and Individual Differences, July 2010
53. Bortz, W. M. 2nd, & Wallace, D. H. (1999). Physical fitness, aging, and sexuality. Western Journal of Medicine, 170, 167-175.
54. Penhollow, T et al; Sexual Desirability and Sexual Performance: Does Exercise and Fitness Really Matter? Electronic Journal of Human Sexuality, Volume 7, October 5, 2004
55. Lorenz, TA et al; EXERCISE IMPROVES SEXUAL FUNCTION IN WOMEN TAKING ANTIDEPRESSANTS: RESULTS FROM A RANDOMIZED CROSSOVER TRIAL; Depress Anxiety. 2014 Mar; 31(3): 188–195.
56. Binks et al; Duke University findings presented on Nov. 15, 2004, at the annual meeting of The North American Association for the Study of Obesity
57. Babraj, J et al; The impact of brief high-intensity exercise on blood glucose levels; Diabetes Metab Syndr Obes. 2013; 6: 113–122.

58. Geda, et al; Physical Exercise and Mild Cognitive Impairment: A Population-Based Study; Arch Neurol. 2010 Jan. 67 (1) 80-86.
59. Golomb, BA; A Fat to Forget: Trans Fat Consumption and Memory; PLOS One; Published: June 17, 2015
60. University of California, Los Angeles (UCLA), Health Sciences. "High-fructose diet slows recovery from brain injury." ScienceDaily. 2 October 2015.
61. Smyth et al; Healthy eating and reduced risk of cognitive declineAmerican Academy of Neurology; Neurology; May 6, 2015
62. Farah NMF, Gill JMR; Effects of Exercise Before or After Meal Ingestion on fat balance and postprandial digestion; British Journal of Nutrition. Published online October 26 2012
63. Atkinson, G et al; Chronobiological considerations for exercise and heart disease; Sports Med, 2006;36(6):487-500.
64. Scurr, J et al; Breast Displacement in Three Dimensions During the Walking and Running Gait Cycle; Journal of Applied Biomechanics, 2009, 25, 322-329
65. Paul T. Williams and Paul D. Thompson. Walking Versus Running for Hypertension, Cholesterol, and Diabetes Mellitus Risk Reduction. Arteriosclerosis, Thrombosis and Vascular Biology, April 4 2013
66. Pocari, J et al; Fitness and weight loss when walking with poles; ACE magazine, 1997
67. Yates et al; Association between change in daily ambulatory activity and cardiovascular events in people with impaired glucose tolerance (NAVIGATOR trial): a cohort analysis; The Lancet; Vol 383, no 9922 p1059–1066, 22 March 2014
68. Kosmadakis et al; Benefits of regular walking exercise in advanced pre-dialysis chronic kidney disease; Nephrol. Dial. Transplant 2012 Mar;27(3):997-1004.
69. Williams, P; National Runners Health Study; presented at the 69th Scientific Sessions of the American Heart Association, 1996
70. Duck-chul Lee et al; Aerobics Center Longitudinal Study (ACLS); presented at the American College of Sports Medicine 2012 Annual Meeting
71. Williams, PT; Effects of running and walking on osteoarthritis and hip replacement risk; Med.Sci. Sorts. Exerc.;2013 Jul;45(7):1292-7.
72. Fries et al; Reduced disability and mortality among aging runners: a 21-year longitudinal study; Arch intern Med; 2008 Aug 11;168(15):1638-46.
73. Moore, I; RUNNING SELF-OPTIMISATION: ACUTE AND SHORT-TERM ADAPTATIONS TO RUNNING MECHANICS AND RUNNING ECONOMY; Exeter University July 2013
74. Anderson, LB et al; All-Cause Mortality Associated With Physical Activity During Leisure Time, Work, Sports, and Cycling to Work; Jama Internal Medicine; June 12 2000, Vol 160 (11)
75. Pollock RD, Carter S, Velloso CP, Duggal NA, Lord JM, Lazaraus NR, Harridge SDR; An investigation into the relationship between age and physiological function in highly active older adults; published online in The Journal of Physiology on Tuesday 6 January 2015.
76. Burgomaster et al; Similar metabolic adaptations during exercise after low volume sprint interval and traditional endurance training in humans; J.Physiol; 2008 Jan 1;586(1):151-60.
77. Sim AY et al; High-intensity intermittent exercise attenuates ad-libitum energy intake; Int J Obes.; 2014 Mar;38(3):417-22
78. Babraj et al; High intensity training improves health and physical function in middle aged adults; Biology; 2014 May 12;3(2):333-44.

79. Babraj JA, Vollaard NB, Keast C, Guppy FM, Cottrell G, Timmons JA (2009) Extremely short duration high intensity interval training substantially improves insulin action in young healthy males. BMC Endocr Disord. 9: 1-8

80. Olson, M; Four minute workout routine; 60th annual conference of the American College of Sports Medicine 2013

81. Hutchins, K; Nautilus funded Osteoporosis Study at the University of Florida (1982- 1986)

82. Westcott,WL; Effects of regular and slow speed resistance training on muscle strength; Journal of Sports Medicine and Physical Fitness 2001 Jun;41(2):154-8.

83. Gothe, NP et al; The effects of an 8-week Hatha yoga intervention on executive function in older adults. J Gerentol A Biol Sci Med Sci; 2014 Sep;69(9):1109-16.

84. Loughren, E.A. (2010). Motivation of first time marathoners to adherence to marathoning. Dissertation Abstracts International: Section B: The Sciences and Engineering, 70, 9-B

85. ACSM; 2012 The Motivation to Exercise

86. Hunter GR et al; Combined aerobic and strength training and energy expenditure in older women. Med.Sci Sports. Exerc; 2013 Jul;45(7):1386-93.

87. Kell et al; The influence of periodized resistance training on strength changes in men and women. J Strength Cond Res; 2011 Mar;25(3):735-44.

88. Chowdhury et al; Association of dietary, circulating, and supplement fatty acids with coronary risk: a systematic review and meta-analysis. Ann Intern Med; 2014 Mar 18;160(6):398-406.

89. Stote et al; A controlled trial of reduced meal frequency without caloric restriction in healthy, normal-weight, middle-aged adults; Am J Clin Nutr. Author manuscript; available in PMC 2009 Feb 20.

90. Oscar H. Franco, Yim Lun Wong, Jane E Ferrie et al; Cross-cultural Comparison of Correlates of Quality of Life and Health Status: The Whitehall II Study (UK) and the Western New York Health Study (US); European Journal of Epidemiology, March 2012

91. Steptoe et al; Positive affect measured using ecological momentary assessment and survival in older men and women; Proceedings of the National Academy of Sciences of the USA vol. 108 no. 45 18244–18248, d

92. Madssen et al; Peak Oxygen Uptake after Cardiac Rehabilitation: A Randomized Controlled Trial of a 12-Month Maintenance Program versus Usual Care; PLoS One. 2014; 9(9):

93. Meier; Validity of consumer-based physical activity monitors.Med.Sci. Sports.Exerc; 2014 Sep;46(9):1840-8.

94. Devor; Mammalian Skeletal Tissue Response to Exercise; journal Applied Physiology March 2005

95. Mutrie et al; Behavior change techniques used to promote walking and cycling: a systematic review; Health Psychology, vol 32, no. 8, pp. 1-11.

96. Yates et al; Association between change in daily ambulatory activity and cardiovascular events in people with impaired glucose tolerance (NAVIGATOR trial): a cohort analysis, The Lancet 20 December 2013

97. Yaffe, K et al; A prospective study of physical activity and cognitive decline in elderly women: women who walk. Arch Intern Med; 2001 Jul 23;161(14):1703-8.

98. Law, RY et al; Warm-up reduces delayed onset muscle soreness but cool-down does not: a randomised controlled trial. Aust J Physio; 2007;53(2):91-5.

Index

abs exercises
    basics 237
    crunches 237–8
    knee crossovers 239–40
    oblique crunches 238–9
    plank 238
    Russian twists 240
    side plank 240
    Superman 238
    V-sits 239
activity 81–4
ageing
    causes of 32–4
    effects of 13–20
    nature/nurture 34–9
alcohol 252–3
antioxidants 69–70, 100, 109–10, 112

back fat 15–16
barre workouts 243–4
basal metabolic rate (BMR) 51–2
bingo wings 19–20
blood sugar levels 62, 67, 82, 99–100, 115
bone health 43, 45–8, 85, 111, 212, 225
boob droopage 18–19
breakfast 9, 53–7, 106

calisthenics 79–80, 175
    alternate lunges 234
    basics 231–2
    chair dips 236
    lateral lunges 236–7
    push-ups 232–3
    single body leg lifts 234–5
    squats 233
    step-ups 235–6
    sumo squats 233–4
    walking lunges 234
    wall squats 235
calories 9, 22–4, 51–3, 61, 83, 86, 87, 115, 219, 220
cankles 17
carbohydrates 66–7, 247–8
cardio 174
    basics 210–11
    cycling 215, 255–6
    rowing 216–17
    running 213–15
    swimming 215–16
    walking 211–13, 254–5
cheat days 256
cognitive function 100–1
cool-downs 255–6
cycling 215, 255–6

delayed onset muscle soreness (DOMS) 253
diabetes 23–4, 43, 62, 63, 82, 211–12
diet plan 107–12
    how to eat 107–8
    progression 241–2
    shopping list - week 1: 138–9
    shopping list - week 2: 150–1
    shopping list - week 3: 162–3
    shopping list - week 4: 169–70
    storecupboard ingredients - week 1: 139–40
    storecupboard ingredients - week 2: 151–2

storecupboard ingredients - week 3: 164
storecupboard ingredients - week 4: 169–70
tips 117
weekly plans 123–6
what to avoid 121
what to eat 109–12
what to expect 115–17
what's allowed 122
dumbbells 175–6

equipment 175–8
exercise guidelines 77–84
exercise plan 112–14
cardio intensity 173–4
day 1: 180
day 2: 181
day 3: 182
day 4: 183
day 5: 184
day 6: 185
day 7: 186
day 8: 187
day 9: 188
day 10: 189
day 11: 190
day 12: 191
day 13: 192
day 14: 193
day 15: 194
day 16: 195
day 17: 196
day 18: 197
day 19: 198
day 20: 199
day 21: 200
day 22: 201
day 23: 202
day 24: 203
day 25: 204
day 26: 205
day 27: 206
day 28: 207
day 29: 208
day 30: 209
how to exercise 114
progression 242–3
tips 118–19
what it entails 172–3
what to expect 115–17
when to exercise 112–13, 172
where to start 171–2
exercises, see abs exercises; calisthenics; cardio; short HIIT; weight burners

facial fat loss 90–1, 92
fascia 80
fasting 22–4, 57–9, 62–5, 107, 118, 249
fat (body fat) 17, 18, 85–6, 88
fat (dietary fat) 67, 110–11, 248–9
fitness age 26–7
fitness, decline in 84–9
fitness-fasting 57–9, 118
fitness language 173–5
fitness trackers 252
flexibility 80
food diaries 106–7
4-hour fast 62–5, 107, 249
free radicals 33, 69
fruit 25, 67, 111–12, 248

glucose 63–4
goal-setting 245–6
grazing 59–62
gym balls 178
gym face 90–1, 92

happiness 249
hatha yoga 243
heart health 95–6, 251
HIIT (high intensity interval training) 174–5, 251
long HIIT 174, 217–18
short HIIT 175, 219–24

hormones
    cortisol   18, 41, 81
    effects of disruption   15, 17,
        18–19, 20, 39–42
    glucagon   64
    human growth hormone
        (HGH)   81
    insulin   37, 58, 63–4, 99
    insulin-like growth factor 1
        (IGF-1)   23, 64–5
    oestrogen   17, 18, 40–1, 45, 91
    progesterone   18
hunger   10, 246
    dealing with   250

inactivity, effects of   82
insulin resistance   18, 43, 101
intensity   77–8

joint health   96–8, 212

knees   16–17
kyphosis   49, 88

libido   98–9
lipolysis   63
long HIIT   174, 217–18

meal composition   65–9
meal times   106–7
men, ageing in   20
menopause   17, 39, 40, 41–2
metabolic syndrome   63–4, 96
metabolism   4, 9, 20, 24, 41, 43,
        51–2
motivation   244–6
muscle mass   20, 23–4, 41, 42–5, 88

ORAC (oxygen radical absorbency
        capacity) scores   69–70
osteoarthritis   16–17, 96–8, 214
osteopenia   45
osteoporosis   43, 45–6, 49, 88, 225
oxidation   33, 69

perimenopause   18, 40, 41
phytoestrogens   110
posture: exercises   48–9
protein   67
ptosis   18–19

recipes - week   1
    apple and pork meatballs in a spicy
        tomato sauce   134–5
    berry porridge   128
    buckwheat pancakes with
        cherries   128–9
    chicken, avocado, apple and
        hazelnut salad   131
    chicken, butternut squash and
        baby sweetcorn stir fry   132–3
    crab and avocado lettuce
        wrap   131–2
    curried carrot and chickpea
        soup   130
    halloumi kebabs with watermelon
        and feta salad   135–6
    lamb tagine with jewelled
        quinoa   136–7
    lemony prawns with white
        beans   133
    oat berry smoothie   127
    skinny mackerel kedgeree   129–30
    turkey mince and kidney bean
        chilli   137–8
recipes - week   2
    beef and Jerusalem artichoke
        stew   148
    Brazil nut dip   143–4
    butternut squash and chickpea
        salad   143
    date and rice porridge   141–2
    kale and red lentil soup   142
    lime and coriander chicken with
        Puy lentils   148–50
    spicy chicken and radish
        salad   146
    spicy eggs   140–1

tofu stir fry 144–5
tuna steak with spicy mango
    salsa 145
turkey and apricot meatballs with
    bulgur wheat 146–7
recipes - week 3
    avocado hash 153–4
    baked pistachio chicken with sugar
        snap peas 158
    beetroot, feta and orange
        salad 156–7
    citrus salmon 161–2
    crab cakes 159–60
    crushed new potatoes with mackerel
        and mushrooms 154–5
    French fish stew 160
    lamb with barley 161
    nut and bean tabbouleh 157
    pepper frittata 152–3
    pork stir fry 159
    spicy sweetcorn chowder 155
recipes - week 4
    chicken and butterbean
        salad 167–8
    chicken soba noodles 168–9
    grilled fruit 164–5
    muffin stack 165
    pea dip 166–7
    prawn pho 166
    salsa verde 168
recovery 80–1
resistance exercise 44, 46–7
Rev5: 243

sarcopenia 42–5
short HIIT 175, 219–24
    basics 219–20
    burpees 221
    high knee sprints 222
    indoor cycle sprints 224
    jump squats 223
    jumping jacks 223
    mountain climbers 222

spotty dogs 221–2
squat thrusts 223–4
stair climbing 220–1
sleep 41, 81, 113, 116–17
sports bras 177–8
stopwatches 176
stress 18, 41, 81, 243
stretching 80, 114, 243
sugar 24–5
supplements 254

10 commandments 246–9
thermogenesis 51–2
trainers 176
treadmill classes 244
twin studies 35–9

VO$_2$ max 26

walking 211–13, 254–5
waterproof clothing 176–7
weight burners
    Arnold press 227–8
    basics 224
    bent over row 230–1
    bicep curls 230
    lateral raises 227
    reverse fly 228
    shoulder press 226
    single arm fly 226–7
    triceps kickbacks 228–9
    triceps overhead extensions 225–6
    upright row 230
    weighted calf raises 229
    weighted side bends 229–30
    wood chopper 231
weight gain 41, 42, 63
weight loss 10
weight loss plateau 252
weight training 78–9, 247

yoga 80, 243